关爱健康

Liebe die Gesundheit

Love Your Health

丁宏余
Ding HongYu

# 关爱健康
# Liebe die Gesundheit
# Love Your Health

## 新八段锦
## Die Neuen Acht Brokate
## The New Eight Brocades

## 拉筋正骨功
## Sehnen- und Knochen-QiGong
## QiGong of the Sinews and Bones

珍惜生命　Schätze das Leben　Cherish Your Life

# 版本说明

作者　丁宏余教授
编辑发行　Alexander Callegari

翻译
中德翻译:　宋焱 Yan Gronau
德英翻译:　Heide-Marie Hönow

校对　Dr. Jürgen Geuder，Yan Gronau，Heide-Marie Hönow

版面设计　Alexander Callegari

照片和图样　Alexander Callegari，Maximilian Callegari，丁宏余教授，Richard Geitner


2015年第一版
ISBN 978-3-934785-75-5



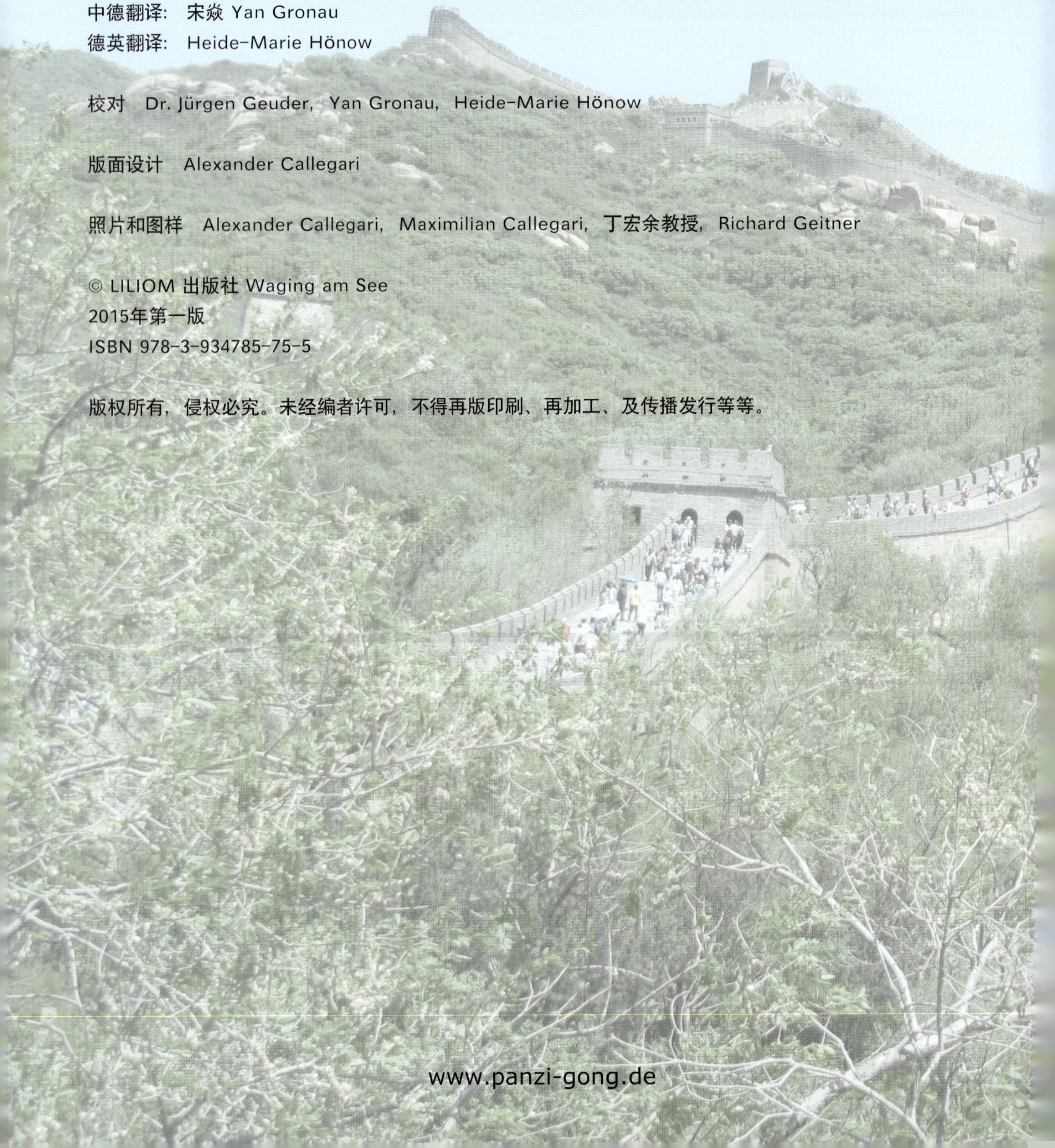

www.panzi-gong.de

# Impressum

Autor: Professor Ding HongYu
Herausgeber: Alexander Callegari

Übersetzung: Chinesisch - Deutsch Yan Gronau; Deutsch - Englisch Heide-Marie Hönow

Lektorat: Dr. Jürgen Geuder, Yan Gronau und Heide-Marie Hönow

Layout: Alexander Callegari
Fotos/Zeichnungen: Alexander und Maximilian Callegari, Prof. Ding HongYu, Richard Geitner


1. Auflage 2015
ISBN 978-3-934785-75-5



# Imprint

Author: Professor Ding HongYu
Editor: Alexander Callegari

Translation: Chinese - German Yan Gronau; German - English Heide-Marie Hönow

Proof Reading: Dr. Jürgen Geuder, Yan Gronau and Heide-Marie Hönow

Layout: Alexander Callegari
Photos/Drawings: Alexander and Maximilian Callegari, Prof. Ding HongYu, Richard Geitner


1st edition 2015
ISBN 978-3-934785-75-5



www.panzi-gong.de

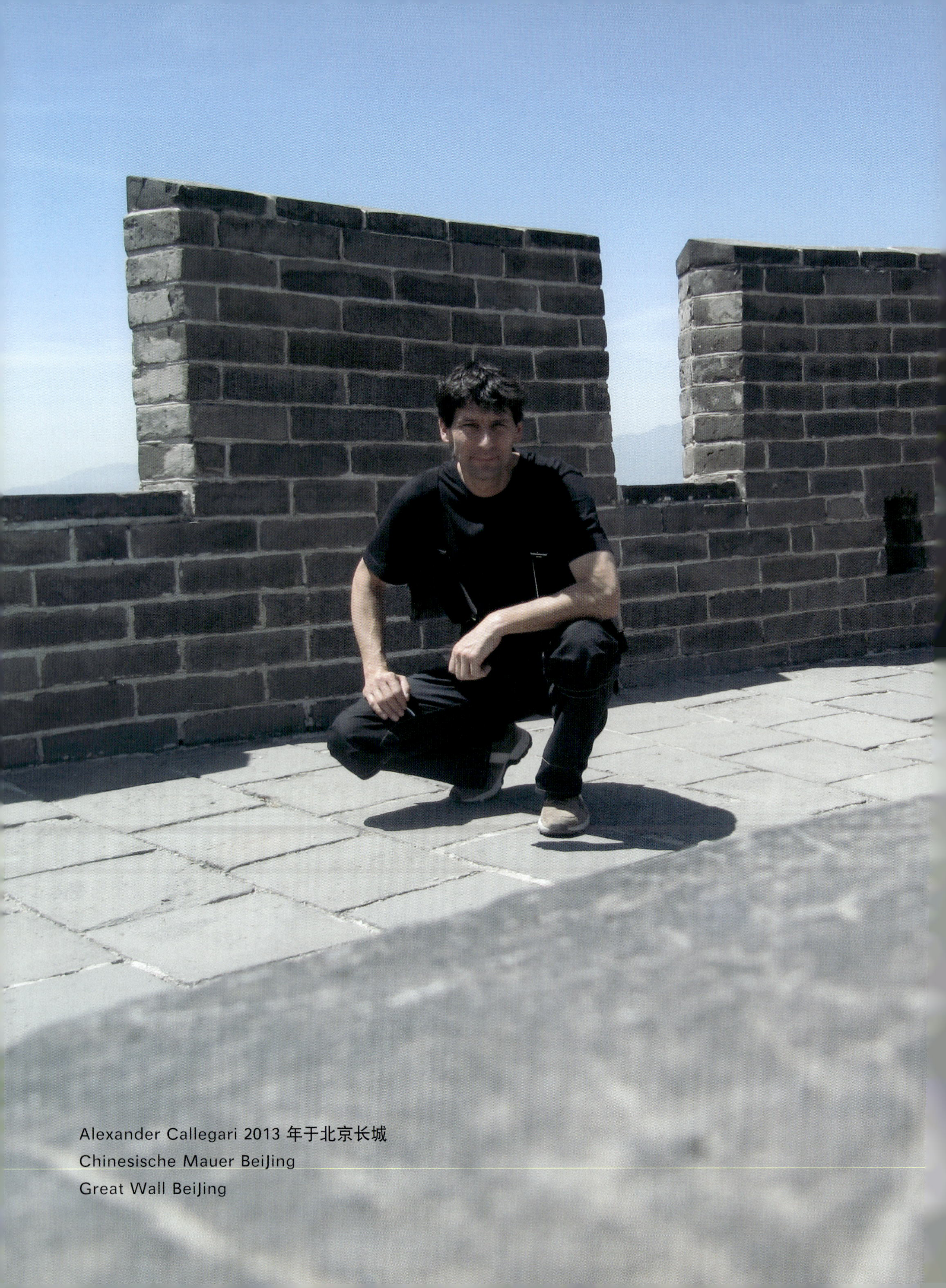

Alexander Callegari 2013 年于北京长城
Chinesische Mauer BeiJing
Great Wall BeiJing

# 目录

## Inhaltsverzeichnis

# Table of Contents

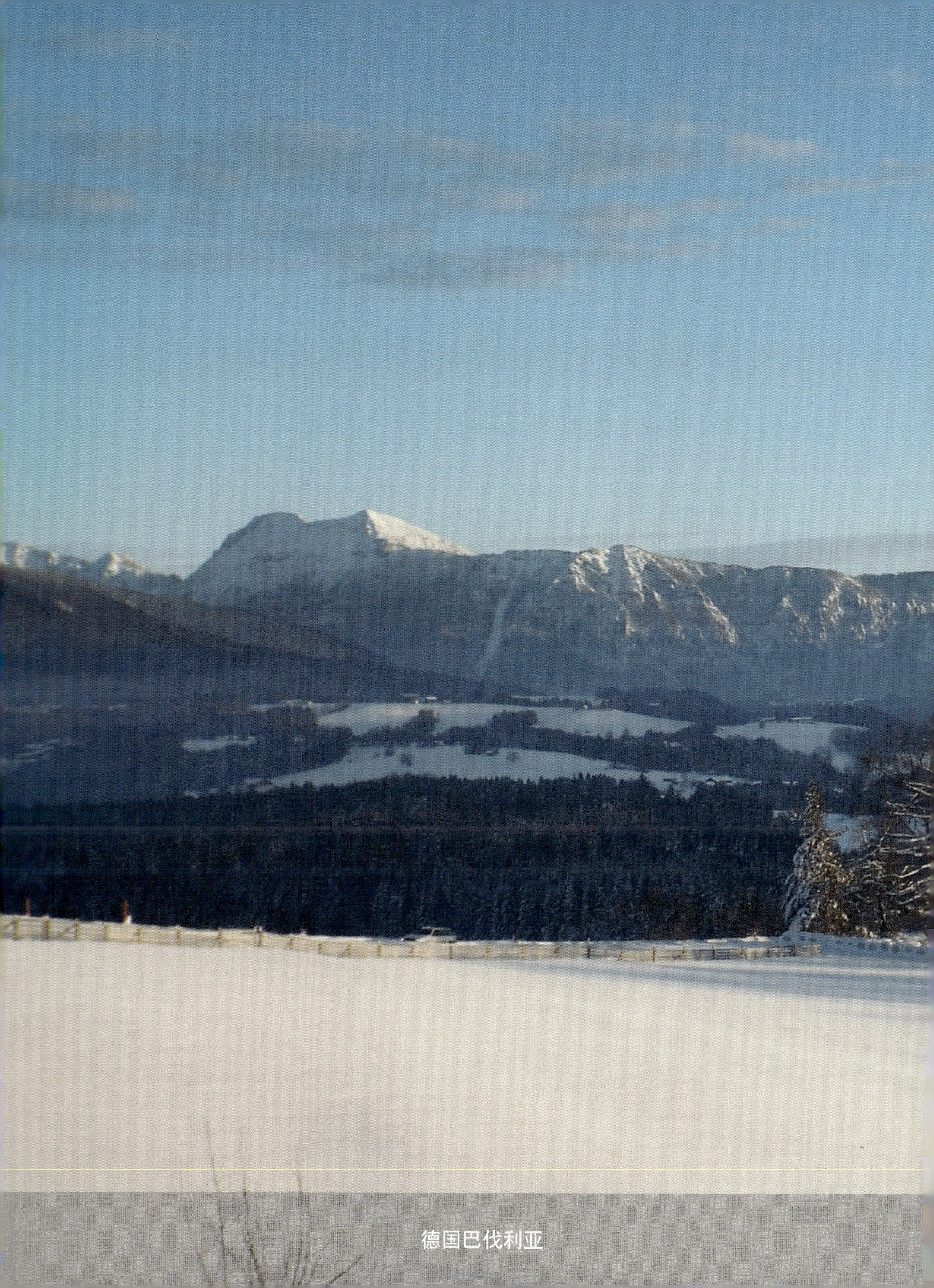

德国巴伐利亚

Bayern Deutschland

Bavaria Germany

# 序言

1996年秋天，我有幸认识了来自南京大学的丁宏余教授。丁教授当时已在南京大学体育系教授了很多年太极拳、气功及武术。在德国访问期间，他想找一家合适的机构，以便开授太极拳和气功课程，让中国的太极和气功在德国得到更为广泛的传播。他的这个想法和 Mettnau 疗养院当时通过体育锻炼，使病人能够更快康复的构想不谋而合。Mettnau 疗养院坐落于博登湖旁，是德国有名的医护疗养中心，我在那里是体育部的教练和负责人。

就这样，从1996年起，丁教授每年在 Mettnau 教授医疗保健气功和太极拳。2000年在 Mettnau 发起了“Mettnau 太极和气功日”，这个项目一直到2007年都是由丁教授亲自带领。不仅 Mettnau 的疗养病人从丁教授的课程中学到了健康体育的知识，我也从中得益匪浅。从此中国传统的太极和气功在 Mettnau 一直作为常规课开设，很多人康复后，还专门回到 Mettnau 参加丁教授的课程。2007年后，丁教授由于年龄原因不再来访德国，我作为他的学生继续把“Mettnau 太极和气功日”一直办到今天。

我和丁教授自1996年一直到现在都有联系。我曾分别于2001年和2006年到中国拜访过丁教授。Alexander Callegari 先生不仅是我在太极和气功上志同道合的好朋友，也和我一样是丁教授的学生。让我十分敬佩的是，他除了多年来勤奋认真的钻研和学习太极拳、气功、武术外，还不断的把丁宏余教授创编的功法和养生保健的练习以直观的、一目了然的形式出版成书。

太极拳和气功是一项由来已久的人类自我养生保健的活动，是中国古老文化的遗产，是中国人民几千年来在自身锻炼调理的实践中，逐步积累经验和理论而发展起来的一项运动。Alexander Callegari 这次编辑的第二本丁宏余教授的功法练习给许多太极和气功爱好者带来了福音和新的体验。我也希望这本书作为教科书能继续传承下去。

Richard Geitner
Mettnau 疗养院体育部和理疗部主任，太极拳和气功教练
2015年2月
于德国 Radolfzell

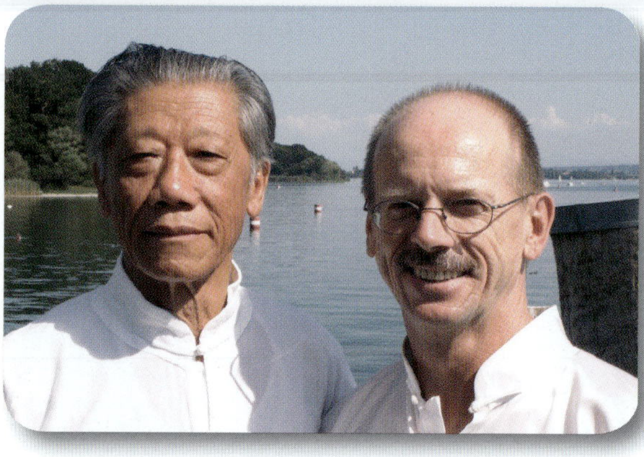

丁宏余教授 – Richard Geitner 2006年

# 编者前言

我很高兴在这里能再次推出丁宏余教授编创的第二部功法练习。丁宏余教授退休前曾在南京大学体育系执教近四十年。通过他长期对太极拳、气功及武术的研究和实践经验，编创了许多新的气功、太极功法。自1988年起，先后应奥登堡大学、德国气功协会和 Mettnau 疗养院等单位的邀请，他14次来访德国开授课程，为中西方体育文化交流作出了贡献。
1991年他演练的“大雁气功”在德国西南无线电视台播出；1995年丁教授编创了“五脏气功”；1996年新编“八段锦”；在后面的几年里，丁教授又陆续创编了“保健气功二”和“转盘健身功”。2012年和2014年又编写了“拉筋正骨功”和“老人延寿十八法”两个保健练习功法。
本书作为教科书编有其中的“新编八段锦”和“拉筋正骨功”两个健身练习。除中文原文外还附加有详细图解以及对几个重要穴位、手式和基本步型的注解。

在此我感谢丁宏余教授多年来对我的帮助和支持，以及为我编辑此书提供的大量文字资料和图片。感谢 Yan Gronau（宋焱女士）对本书作的中德翻译及提出的良好建议。感谢 Heide-Marie Hönow 女士将本书译成英文文本，并对编辑稿件和校对做出很大帮助。Jürgen Geuder 医生是这本书的医学顾问，并对文稿纠正和编辑做了大量工作。感谢 Mettnau 疗养院体育部的负责人 Richard Geitner 先生对此书的关注和多年来对我的大力支持。感谢我的家人 Gabriele、Sandra、Maximilian 对我的耐心、鼓励，和对本书提供的照片摄影和宝贵意见。谢谢大家！
最后我祝愿大家通过练习此书中的功法身体健康，心情舒畅，精神愉快。

Alexander Callegari
2015年2月
于德国 Traunstein

## Vorwort

Im Herbst 1996 kam es zu meiner schicksalhaften Begegnung mit Professor Ding HongYu, einem chinesischen QiGong- und TaiJi-Lehrer aus NanJing in Zentralchina. Während eines Deutschlandaufenthaltes suchte er geeignete Institutionen, um seinen QiGong-Unterricht einem interessierten Publikum vorzustellen. Das passte genau zum Konzept der Mettnau-Kur, einer medizinischen Reha-Einrichtung der Stadt Radolfzell/Bodensee. Es ist eines der bedeutendsten und traditionsreichsten Zentren für Bewegungstherapie in Deutschland, in dem ich als Sportlehrer tätig war und heute noch bin.
Mit Professor Ding hatte ich einen Lehrer ersten Ranges, der mich in meinem Streben nach therapiegeeigneten QiGong-Formen tatkräftigt unterstützte. Medizinisches QiGong des modernen China, aber auch alte traditionelle Formen des QiGong und TaiJi Quan wurden auf der Mettnau etabliert und finden bis heute viele Anhänger und Freunde. Diese Entwicklung hat Professor Ding mit jährlichen Seminaren vor Ort in Radolfzell/Deutschland seit 1996 begleitet. Im Jahr 2000 wurden die „Mettnau TaiJi und QiGong Tage" ins Leben gerufen, die Professor Ding bis 2007 persönlich leitete. Seitdem führe ich die Seminare weiter, nachdem Professor Ding sich entschlossen hat, nicht mehr zu reisen. 2001 und 2006 konnte ich während zweier Chinaaufenthalte den Kontakt zu Professor Ding weiter pflegen.

Alexander Callegari – meinem langjährigen guten Freund und Mitstreiter in Sachen QiGong – gebührt höchstes Lob und Anerkennung, dass er die guten Kontakte zu unserem gemeinsamen Lehrer nicht abreißen ließ – ja sie sogar noch forcierte, indem er die von Professor Ding entwickelten QiGong-Formen in sehr anschaulicher Art und Weise zu Papier gebracht und herausgegeben hat.
Mit diesem zweiten Buch hat Professor Ding HongYu zusammen mit dem Herausgeber Alexander Callegari ein Werk geschaffen, das den vielen QiGong-Interessierten nicht nur große Freude bereiten wird, sondern auch eine Bereicherung der medizinischen Bewegungsformen darstellt und Lehrbuch für künftige Generationen sein kann.

Richard Geitner
Bereichsleiter Sport- und Physiotherapie, TaiJi- und QiGonglehrer
Radolfzell, Februar 2015
Deutschland

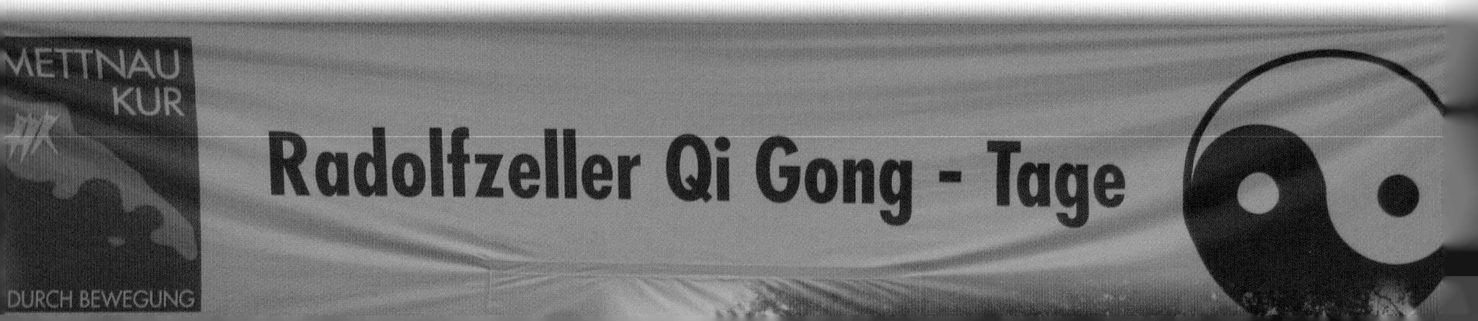

# Vorwort

Es freut mich sehr, Ihnen das zweite Buch über QiGong Formen meines Lehrers Professor Ding HongYu zu präsentieren. Professor Ding war als TaiJi Quan- und QiGong-Lehrer an der Universität von NanJing der Volksrepublik China tätig. Seit Ende der 50er Jahre beschäftigt er sich mit TaiJi Quan und QiGong und arbeitete in verschiedenen Einrichtungen zur Erforschung der Effekte von TaiJi Quan und QiGong.
Seit 1988 war er 14 Mal in Deutschland, wurde u. a. von der Universität Oldenburg, dem Deutschen QiGong Verein und der Mettnau Kur eingeladen, um Kurse und Seminare abzuhalten. Er hat dadurch zum Kulturaustausch zwischen Ost und West beigetragen.
1991 war er an der Verfilmung des Lehrprogramms „DaYan („Wildgans") QiGong" beteiligt, das der Südwestfunk Baden-Baden ausstrahlte. 1995 entwickelte Professor Ding das „Fünf Organe QiGong" (WuZang QiGong), 1996 modifizierte er die Form der „Acht Brokatstücke" (BaDuanJin). Im folgenden Jahr entwickelte er das „Gesundheitsschützende QiGong 2" (BaoJian QiGong 2) und 1998 die Form der „Gesundheitsübung mit der Tellerdrehung"[1] (PanZi Gong - Teller Gong). 2012 entwickelte er das „Sehnen- und Knochen-QiGong" (JinGu Gong) und 2014 die „Lebensverlängernden Übungen" (LaoRen YanShou Fa).
Im vorliegenden Buch finden Sie zwei Formen, eine klassische Form mit langer Tradition, die „Acht Brokatstücke" und die Form des Sehnen- und Knochen-QiGongs. Das Buch ist als Übungsbuch konzipiert. Neben einer genauen Darstellung der Formen finden Sie die chinesischen Originaltexte sowie im Anhang die Hand- und Fußstellungen, Erklärungen zu Fachbegriffen und Akupunkturpunkten.

Alexander Callegari
Traunstein, Februar 2015
Deutschland

Mein herzlicher Dank gilt:
Professor Ding HongYu für sein Vertrauen, mir dieses Material zur Veröffentlichung zu geben; Yan Gronau (geb. Song) für ihre Übersetzungsarbeit der chinesischen Originaltexte, ihre Meinung, ihre guten Ratschläge und ihre Unterstützung; Heide-Marie Hönow, die ihre Ideen beisteuerte, das Manuskript redigierte und Korrektur las, sowie für ihre Übersetzung der deutschen Texte ins Englische; Dr. Jürgen Geuder für die Klärung der medizinischen Aspekte und seine Lektorarbeit; Richard Geitner, dem sportlichen Leiter der Mettnau-Kur/Radolfzell, für seine jahrelange Unterstützung und Freundschaft; meiner Frau Gabriele, meiner Tochter Sandra und meinem Sohn Maximilian für ihre Unterstützung, Meinungen, Ideen und Fotografiearbeit.

---

[1] Zu dieser Form ist 2012 ein Übungsbuch in vier Sprachen (Chinesisch, Deutsch, Englisch, Französisch) unter dem Titel „Gesundheitsübung mit der Tellerdrehung" im LILIOM Verlag Waging erschienen. ISBN 978-3-934785-60-1.

# Foreword

In the autumn of 1996 I had my providential encounter with Professor Ding HongYu, a Chinese teacher of QiGong- and TaiJi from NanJing in Central China. During a stay in Germany he was looking for an adequate institution to present his QiGong training to an interested audience. This fit exactly into the concept of Mettnau-Kur, medical institution for rehabilitation of the town of Radolfzell/Bodensee. It is one of the most important and traditional centres for movement therapy in Germany, where I have been working as a physical instructor up to the present day. In Professor Ding I had a first-rate teacher who supported me energetically in my striving for therapy-suited QiGong forms. Medical QiGong of modern China as well as traditional forms of QiGong and TaiJi were established in Mettnau-Kur and have found many disciples and friends up to this very day. Professor Ding has accompanied this development with yearly seminars in Radolfzell/Germany since 1996. In the year 2000 the "Mettnau TaiJi and QiGong Days" were created and presided by Professor Ding personally up to 2007. Since then I carry on the seminars after Professor Ding decided to travel no longer. 2001 and 2006 I was able to further my contact with Professor Ding during two stays in China.

To Alexander Callegari – my good friend of long years and partner in striving in the field of QiGong – my highest praise and appreciation is due for keeping up the good contacts with our common teacher and even enforcing them by writing down and editing in a very clear manner the QiGong forms developed by Professor Ding.
In this second book Professor Ding HongYu together with editor Alexander Callegari has created a publication which will not only give great pleasure to many people interested in QiGong, but will also enrich medical forms of movement and can be a book of instruction for coming generations.

Richard Geitner
Director of sport- and physio-therapy, teacher of TaiJi and QiGong
Radolfzell, February 2015
Germany

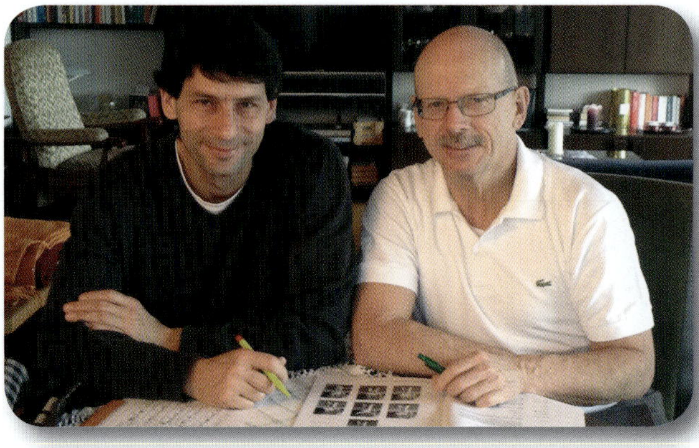

Alexander Callegari - Richard Geitner 2014

# Foreword

I am very happy to present to you the second book on QiGong forms by my teacher Professor Ding HongYu. Professor Ding has been working as a TaiJi- and QiGong teacher at the University of NanJing in the People´s Republic of China. Since the end of the nineteen-fifties he has been engaging in TaiJi Quan and QiGong and has worked in several institutions for the research of the effects of TaiJi Quan and QiGong.
Since 1988 he has paid fourteen visits to Germany and has been invited by Oldenburg University, by the German QiGong Association and Mettnau-Kur, a medical institution for rehabilitation, and by other institutions to hold courses and seminars. Thus he has been attributing to the cultural exchange between east and west.
In 1991 he took part in the making of a film on the teaching program "DaYan ("Wild Goose") QiGong" which was broadcast by Südwestfunk Baden-Baden. In 1995 Professor Ding developed the "Five Organs QiGong" (WuZang QiGong), in 1996 he modified the form of the "Eight Pieces of Brocade" (BaDuanJin). In the following year he developed the "Health-Saving QiGong 2" (BaoJian QiGong 2), and in 1998 the form of the "Health Practice with the Rotation of the Plate"[1] (PanZi Gong - Plate Gong). In 2012 Professor Ding developed the "QiGong of the Sinews and Bones" (JinGu Gong), and in 2014 the "Life-Prolonging Exercises" (LaoRen YanShou Fa).
In the present publication you find two forms, a classical form with a long tradition, the "Eight Pieces of Brocade", and the form of the "QiGong of the Sinews and Bones". The book has been conceived as an exercise book. Apart from an exact description of the forms, you find the original Chinese texts as well as explanations concerning the positions of the hands and feet, notes on technical terms and acupuncture points.

Alexander Callegari
Traunstein, February 2015
Germany

My heartfelt thanks I should like to express to
Professor Ding HongYu for his trusting me with this material for publication. Yan Gronau (née Song) for her work of translating the Chinese originals, her opinions, her good pieces of advice and her support. Heide-Marie Hönow who gave her ideas, revised the manuscript and did the correcting as well as for translating the German text into English. Dr. Jürgen Geuder for his clarification of medical aspects and his lectorate. Richard Geitner, the director of sports at Mettnau-Kur Radolfzell, for his longlasting support and friendship. My wife Gabriele, my daughter Sandra and my son Maximilian for their support, opinions, ideas and photography.

---

[1] In 2012 a book of exercises appeared in four languages (Chinese, German, English, French) with the title "Health Practice with the Rotation of the Plate". LILIOM Verlag Waging, Germany, ISBN 978-3-934785-60-1.

## 南大新编 **八段锦** 丁宏余 编演

按语：八段锦是我国古代的一种健身功法，它有八段动作，故称为八段锦。由于它编排精炼、动作简易、姿势优美、健身却病效果俱佳，所以深受人们的喜爱。

八段锦在民间流传了近千年历史，（有文字记戴已达800余年）它属有氧运动，安全可靠。若单练有针对性，套练有全面性，因此，在体育界、武术界、医学界、气功界，分别用于保健体育、武术功法、医疗体操、健身气功；国家体育总局将《健身气功·八段锦》，列为全民健身运动的内容向全国推广。

《南大新编·八段锦》（下称新八段锦），是我校体育部丁宏余老师，经过十多年的潜心研究和在国内外的教学实践，在传统八段锦各种流派的基础上，保留其精华，增添了新内容，创编了这套《新八段锦》。

它丰富了武术内容，简化了动作名称，加大了动作幅度，减小了运动强度，采用的深吸长呼，提高了供氧量，增添保肾、健脑动作，强化了腿功锻炼…等等，符合运动学和生理学规律，适合于知识分子、老龄同志和慢性病患者练习。起到文人动身练武，老人以柔抗衰，中、青年练功强身。相比之下，《新八段锦》在动作上有所强化，效果上可说是锦上添花，现推荐给广大教职工选练，让老同志提高生活质量，使健康得到延续。

南京大学　　老年体协
2007年2月　退休协会

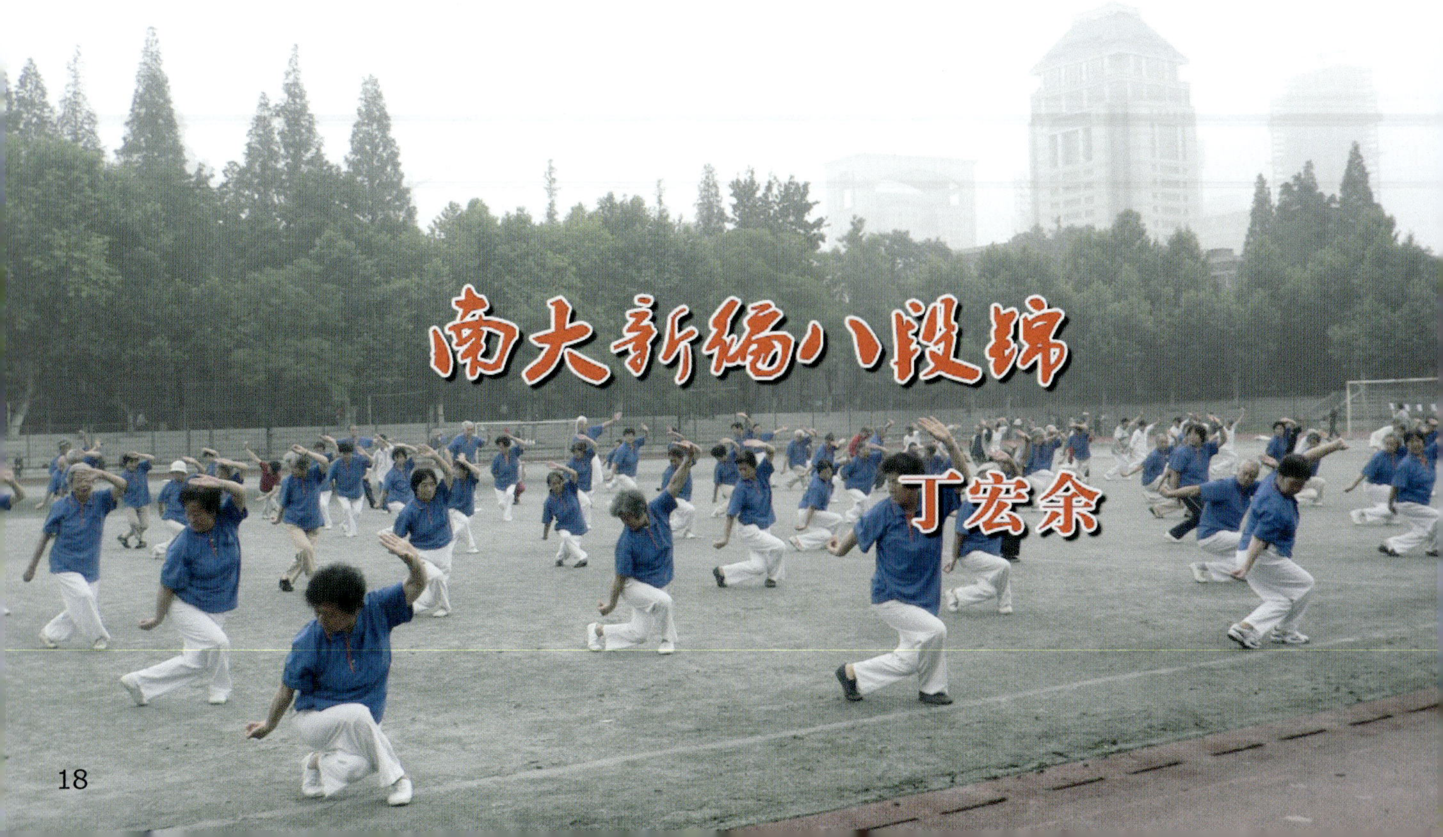

托天理三焦，提神消疲劳。

扩胸强心肺，拉弓似射雕。

单举健脾胃，消化功能好。

转头健大脑，劳伤向后瞧。

摇摆去心火，旋转阴阳调。

要得精气足，躬身固肾腰。

瞪目增气力，聚神出奇效。

放松气血和，七颠诸病消。

# Neues BaDuanJin – Die Neuen Acht Brokate

## Einleitung

Diese neue Fassung wurde kreiert von Professor Ding HongYu von der Universität NanJing[1]. Die folgende Einleitung stammt vom Sportverein für ältere Menschen und Rentner der Universität NanJing, Februar 2007.

BaDuanJin ist eine klassische chinesische Art von Fitness-Übung mit einer langen Tradition. Die Form des BaDuanJin besteht aus acht Übungen. Daraus erklärt sich der Name BaDuanJin: „Acht Stücke Brokat". Wegen der raffinierten Choreographie, einfachen Bewegungen und anmutigen Haltung werden die Übungen mit der Schönheit und Kostbarkeit eines Brokatstoffes gleichgesetzt. Außerdem ist BaDuanJin aufgrund der seit Jahrhunderten bewiesenen positiven Effekte für die Gesundheit bei der Bevölkerung sehr beliebt zur Vorbeugung von Krankheiten. BaDuanJin wurde bereits im 12. Jahrhundert als Text verfasst. In der Überlieferung hat es eine weitaus längere Geschichte.

BaDuanJin ist eine sauerstoffreiche, sichere und zuverlässige Sportart. Die einzelne Übung dient zur Stärkung bestimmter Organe, die komplette Form trainiert den ganzen Körper. In den Bereichen Sport, Kampfkunst, Medizin und QiGong wird BaDuanJin jeweils zur Gesundheitserhaltung, als Kampfsport, zur Krankengymnastik und als Fitness QiQong umfassend praktiziert. Vor über zehn Jahren hat das Chinesische Staatliche Amt für Allgemeinen Sport eine landesweite Kampagne für „gesundheitserhaltendes QiGong und BaDuanJin" als ideale Sportübung für die Förderung der Volksgesundheit durchgeführt.

Die neue Fassung des BaDuanJin der Universität NanJing (wird im Folgenden „Neues BaDuan Jin" genannt) wurde von Professor Ding HongYu, der in der Fachrichtung Sport unserer Universität unterrichtet, neu konzipiert. Mit seiner jahrzehntelangen intensiven Forschung und seiner Unterrichtserfahrung im In- und Ausland, basierend auf einer ganzen Reihe von verschiedenen traditionellen Übungssystemen von BaDuanJin, hat Professor Ding die Übungsformen neu konzipiert. Er hat das Wesentliche beibehalten und neue Inhalte hinzugefügt.

Das Neue BaDuanJin hat den Inhalt der Kampfkunst bereichert und die Namen der Übungen vereinfacht. Die Bewegungsspanne wurde erhöht und die Trainingsbelastung reduziert. Das tiefe Einatmen und lange Ausatmen stehen bewußt im Mittelpunkt der Übungen. Dadurch kommt es zur Verbesserung der Sauerstoffversorgung. Die Beine und die inneren Organe, insbesondere die Nieren, werden gestärkt, die Gehirnfunktion wird aktiviert und vieles mehr.

---

[1] Die Universität von NanJing 南京大学 liegt in der Provinz JiangSu 江苏 im Osten der Volksrepublik China. Die Universität wird kurz auch als NanDa 南大 bezeichnet. In ihrem Ursprung reicht sie bis ins Jahr 258 zurück. Anfang des 20. Jahrhunderts entstand eine moderne Hochschule. Sie gilt als Geburtsstätte der modernen Wissenschaften Chinas und hat im chinesischen Bildungssystem oft eine Vorreiterrolle. Die Universität von NanJing belegt in zahlreichen Rankings immer einen Platz unter den ersten fünf. Sie zählt damit zu den bedeutendsten Universitäten des Landes.

Das Neue BaDuanJin steht im Einklang mit den Gesetzen der Kinematik und Physiologie. Es ist ideal geeignet für Berufstätige mit überwiegend sitzender Tätigkeit, für ältere Menschen – sie können mit den weichen und sanften Bewegungen ihre Beweglichkeit erhalten – und für Menschen mit chronischen Krankheiten. Junge Menschen können durch die Übungen Krankheiten vorbeugen und die Funktionen der inneren Organe stärken. Das Neue BaDuanJin hat die Bewegungen verfeinert und intensiviert. Die Übungseffekte wurden nochmals erhöht. Daher ist das Neue BaDuanJin für die breite Bevölkerung sehr zu empfehlen, da es die Lebensqualität verbessert und die Gesundheit fördert.

## Lyrik[1] des Neuen BaDuanJin

Mit den Händen den Himmel stützen, um den Dreifachen-Erwärmer-Meridian auszurichten.
Die Müdigkeit wird beseitigt und man wird erfrischt.

Das Herz und die Lunge kräftigen.
Die Brust so ausbreiten, als ob man einen Bogen spannt und auf den Geier zielt.

Die Arme einzeln hochheben, um Magen und Milz zu regulieren.
Die Verdauungsfunktion wird angeregt.

Durch Drehungen des Kopfes die Funktionen des Gehirns stärken.
Die von den Fünf Anstrengungen und Sieben Betrübnissen verursachten Krankheiten werden vertrieben.

Mit Wiegen und Wedeln die innere Hitze aus dem Herzen vertreiben.
Yin und Yang werden reguliert.

Die geistige und körperliche Leistungsfähigkeit steigern.
Den Oberkörper tief beugen und die Nieren und den Hüftbereich dadurch stärken.

Die Augen weit öffnen, um die Lebensenergie zu vermehren.
Stärkt und erhöht die Lebensenergie.

Den Körper lockern, um die Energie und das Blut harmonisch auszugleichen.
Sieben Mal den Körper rütteln, hundert Krankheiten vertreiben.

[1] Die chinesische Lyrik unterliegt strengsten Regeln und ist wörtlich nicht übersetzbar. Die obigen Formulierungen geben den Inhalt wieder. Aus der chinesischen Lyrik wurde beibehalten, dass bei den acht Zeilen jeweils im Wechsel der Name bzw. die Wirkungsweise der Übungen zuerst erscheinen.

# New BaDuanJin – The New Eight Brocades

## Introduction

This new version was created by Professor Ding HongYu of NanJing University[1]. The following introduction was given by the sports club for the elderly and retired members of NanJing University in February 2007.

BaDuanJin is a classical Chinese kind of fitness-exercise with a long tradition. BaDuanJin has eight movements, this is why it is called BaDuanJin meaning "Eight Brocades". Because of its refined choreography, the simple movements and the graceful postures, the exercises are compared to the beauty and costliness of brocade fabric. Apart from this BaDuanJin is very popular with the people because of its positive effects for health proven for centuries and prevention of illnesses. As early as in the twelfth century BaDuanJin has been written as a text. In tradition it presumably has a much longer history.
BaDuanJin is a kind of sport rich in oxygen, safe and reliable. The single movement serves the strengthening of specific organs, a complete exercise trains the entire body. In the fields of sport, martial arts, medicine and QiGong BaDuanJin is practised extensively for health keeping, as martial arts sport, for gymnastics for the sick and as fitness QiGong respectively. More than ten years ago the Chinese State Institution for Universal Sport has carried out a country - spanning campaign for "health - preserving QiGong and BaDuanJin" as an ideal sportive exercise for the improvement of the people´s health.

The new version of BaDuanJin from NanJing University (called "New BaDuanJin" in the following text) was freshly created by Professor Ding HongYu who is teaching in the sports department at our university. With his decades – long intensive research and his teaching experience at home and abroad, based on quite a series of various traditional systems of exercise of BaDuanJin, Professor Ding has newly conceived the forms of exercise. He has kept the essentials and added new subject matter.
The New BaDuanJin has enriched the subject matter of martial art and simplified the names of the forms. The span of movement is enhanced and the strain of training is reduced. Breathing in deeply and breathing out a long time deliberately are in the centre of the exercises. They improve the supply of oxygen. Legs and inner organs, especially the kidneys, are strengthened, brain - function is activated and many other effects are brought about.

---

[1] NanJing University 南京大学 is in the province of JiangSu 江苏 in the east of the People´s Republic of China. In short the university is called NanDa 南大. In its origin it goes back as far as 258. In the beginning of the twentieth century the modern university came into existence. It is valued as the birthplace of modern sciences in China and has a leading role in the Chinese system of education. In numerous rankings the University of NanJing always holds a place among the top five. Thus it is one of the most important universities in the country.

New BaDuanJin is in harmony with the laws of kinematics and physiology. It is ideally suited to working people who keep sitting on end in their type of job, for elder people – they may keep their mobility with the help of soft and gentle movements – and chronically ill people. Young people can prevent illnesses by means of the exercise and strengthen the functions of their inner organs. New BaDuanJin has refined the forms and intensified them. The effects of the exercise have once again been enhanced. This is why New BaDuanJin is highly recommendable for the majority of people because it improves the quality of life and is beneficial to your health.

## Lyrics[1] New BaDuanJin

Supporting Heaven with Your Hands, Straighten the Triple-Warmer-Meridian.
Shedding of Tiredness and Being Refreshed.

Your Heart and Lungs Are Strengthened.
Widen Your Chest as if Drawing a Bow to Aim at the Vulture.

Lift Your Arms One by One to Regulate Your Stomach and Your Spleen.
Your Digestive Function Is Stimulated.

Your Brain Functions Are Strengthened by Turnings of Your Head.
Expel the Illnesses Caused by the Five Strains and the Seven Afflictions.

Expel the Inner Heat from Your Heart by Rocking and Wagging.
Yin and Yang Are Regulated.

Your Mental and Bodily Efficiency Is Strengthened.
Bend Your Upper Body Deep Down and Strengthen Your Kidneys and the Region of Your Hips.

Open Your Eyes Wide to Enhance Life Energy.
Strengthens and Enhances Your Life Energy.

Relax Your Body to Balance Your Energy and Blood Harmoniously.
Shaking Seven Times and Expelling a Hundred Illnesses.

[1] Chinese Lyrics are subjected to the most severe rules and cannot be translated word by word. The wordings above represent the contents. From Chinese Lyrics the fact was kept that in the eight lines the name or the function come first alternately.

## 标记注释

a）箭头指出运动方向，用左手臂和左腿做的动作用间断的线条表示，用右手臂和右腿做的动作用不间断的线条表示。用点连成的线条指出头部和腰部的转动方向。箭头结束的地方同时也是下一个动作的开始。重复动作的开始用红色箭头标示。

b）在圆圈内的数字标示动作第几节。它和框架一样，也表示动作段落结束，既一个动作的结束和下一个动作的开始。

a）

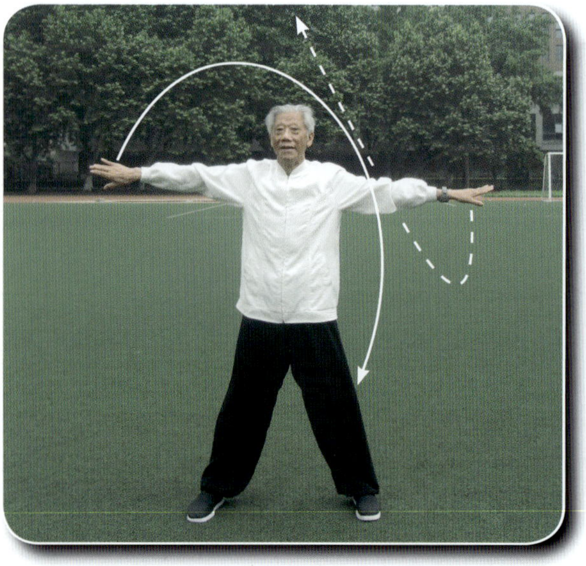

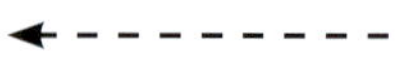

左箭头
links
left

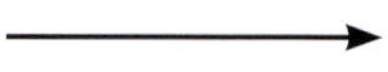

右箭头
rechts
right

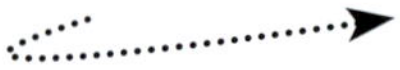

头部和腰部的方向
Kopf-/Hüftrichtung
head/hip direction

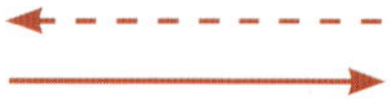

重复
Wiederholung
repetition

## Zeichenerklärungen

a) Die Pfeile geben die Bewegungsrichtungen vor. Die Bewegungen mit dem linken Arm und dem linken Bein sind mit einer gestrichelten Linie dargestellt, die Bewegungen mit rechts mit einer durchgezogenen Linie.
Die Bewegungen des Kopfes und der Hüfte bzw. Taille werden mit einer gepunkteten Linie dargestellt. Das Ende der Pfeilspitze ist immer die Anfangsposition der darauffolgenden Bewegung. Der Anfang einer Wiederholung ist mit roten Pfeilen gekennzeichnet.
b) Die Zahl im Kreis gibt den Bewegungsabschnitt der jeweiligen Übung an. Außerdem zeigt sie, ebenso wie der Rahmen, das Ende eines Bewegungsabschnitts.

## Key to the Symbols Used

a) The arrows show the directions of movement. The movements with the left arm and the left leg are symbolized by a broken line, the movements on the right hand side with an unbroken line.
The movements of the head and the hip and waist respectively are shown with a dotted line. The end of the arrow point always marks the initial position of the following movement. The beginning of a repetition is marked by red arrows.
b) The number in the circle shows the sequence of movement in each exercise. Apart from this the number shows – like the frame – the end of each sequence of movement.

b)

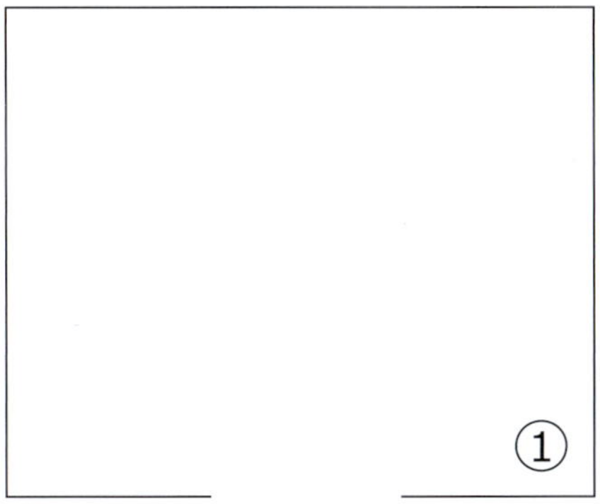


动作段落结束
Ende des Bewegungsabschnitts
end of sequence of movement

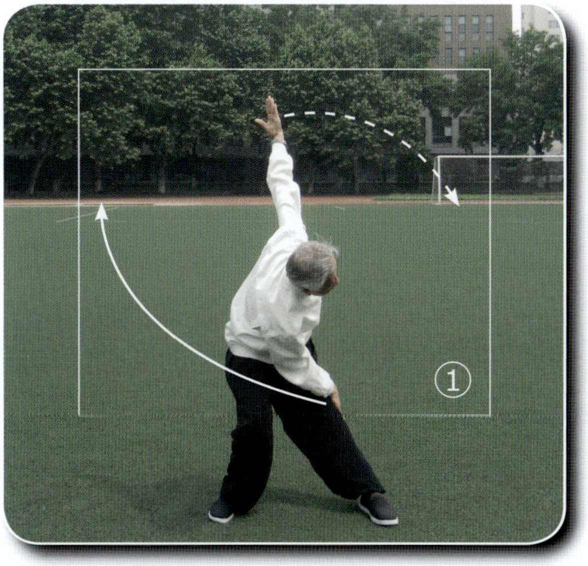

## 练习动作

第一段　托天理三焦

第二段　拉弓似射雕

第三段　单举健脾胃

第四段　劳伤向后瞧

第五段　摇摆去心火

第六段　躬身固肾腰

第七段　瞪目增气力

第八段　七颠诸病消

## Die Übungen

I. Mit den Händen den Himmel stützen und den Dreifachen-Erwärmer-Meridian ausrichten

II. Den Bogen spannen und auf den Geier zielen

III. Die Arme einzeln hochheben, um Magen und Milz zu regulieren

IV. Die von den Fünf Anstrengungen und Sieben Betrübnissen verursachten Krankheiten vertreiben

V. Mit Wiegen und Wedeln die innere Hitze aus dem Herzen vertreiben

VI. Tief beugen, um die Nieren und den Hüftbereich zu stärken

VII. Die Augen weit öffnen – Qi vermehren

VIII. Sieben Mal rütteln und hundert Krankheiten vertreiben

## The Exercises

I. Supporting Heaven with Your Hands, Straighten the Triple-Warmer-Meridian

II. Drawing the Bow and Aiming at the Vulture

III. Lift Your Arms One by One to Regulate Your Stomach and Your Spleen

IV. Expel the Illnesses Caused by the Five Strains and the Seven Afflictions

V. Expel the Inner Heat from Your Heart by Rocking and Wagging

VI. Bend Deep Down to Strengthen Your Kidneys and the Region of Your Hips

VII. Open Your Eyes Wide – Enhancing Qi

VIII. Shaking Seven Times and Expelling a Hundred Illnesses

## 第一段　托天理三焦

预备姿势：上体中正，两脚平行站立，与肩同宽，两臂垂于体侧，两眼平视，舌抵上腭，呼吸自然，周身放松。（图1）

动作

1、吸气时，两手仰掌提至胸前，手指相对，虎口展开。（图2）

2、呼气时，两掌分别向上旋转于肩上，两肘展开，手心向上，手指托耳轮。（图3）

3、吸气时，双手上托至最高限度，掌心向上，虎口相对，眼看前方，同时两足跟提起离地。（图4）

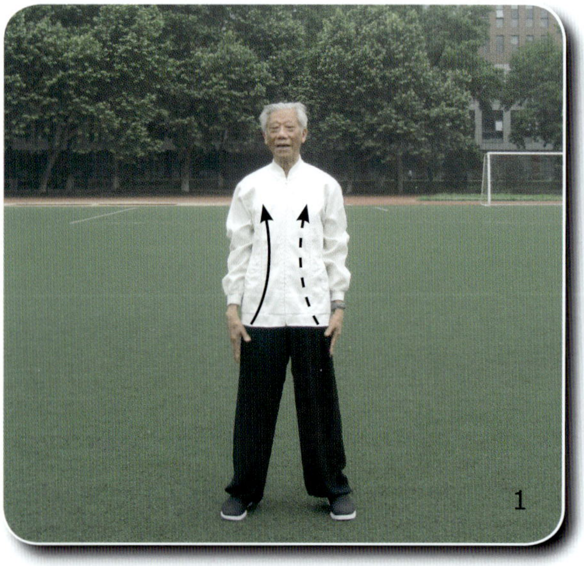

1

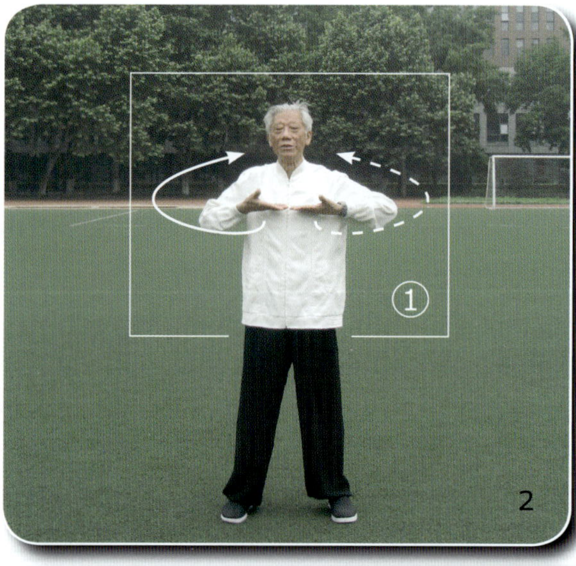


2

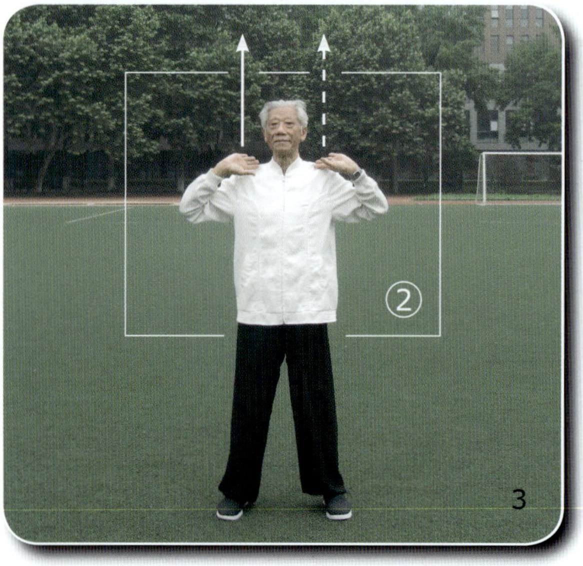


3

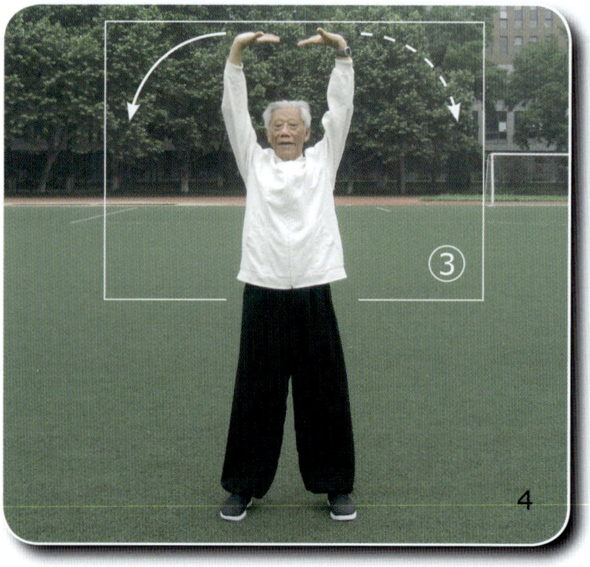


4

## I. Mit den Händen den Himmel stützen und den Dreifachen-Erwärmer-Meridian ausrichten

Ausgangsstellung
Den Oberkörper in eine gerade Position bringen. Die Füße parallel stellen, schulterbreit auseinander. Die Arme hängen an den Seiten des Körpers. Den Blick gerade nach vorne richten. Die Zunge berührt den Gaumen. Natürlich atmen und den ganzen Körper entspannen. Siehe Bild 1.

1. Mit der Einatmung die Hände vor dem Körper von unten nach oben führen bis auf Brusthöhe. Dabei zeigen die Handflächen nach oben, die Fingerspitzen zueinander und der Daumen ist im rechten Winkel abgespreizt. Diese Handposition heißt Tigermaul (HuKou). Siehe Bild 2.
2. Mit der Ausatmung drehen die Hände über die Schulter nach oben. Die Ellenbogen dabei hinaus zu den Seiten schieben, Handflächen nach oben. Am Ende der Bewegung zeigen die Fingerspitzen in Richtung des Halses etwas unterhalb der Ohrläppchen. Siehe Bild 3.
3. Mit der Einatmung die Hände in unveränderter Position so weit wie möglich nach oben strecken. HuKou einander gegenüberstellen. Den Blick nach vorne richten, dabei die Fersen vom Boden lösen. Siehe Bild 4.

## I. Supporting Heaven with Your Hands, Straighten the Triple-Warmer-Meridian

Initial Position
Get the upper part of your body into a straight position. Set your feet parallel, a shoulder breadth apart from each other. Your arms dangle at the sides of your body. Direct your gaze straight ahead of you. Your tongue touches your palate. Breathe naturally and relax your entire body. See illustration 1.

1. While breathing in guide your hands in front of your body from down under upwards to breast height. While doing so your palms point upwards, the tips of your fingers point towards each other and your thumb is spread apart in an angle of 90°. This handposition is called Mouth of the Tiger (HuKou). See illustration 2.
2. While breathing out your hands turn upwards above your shoulders. While doing so shift your elbows outwards to both sides of your body, your palms showing upwards. At the end of the movement your fingertips point in the direction of your neck somewhat beneath your earlobes. See illustration 3.
3. In breathing in stretch your hands as far up as possible keeping your position unchanged. Position HuKou opposite each other. Direct your gaze ahead of you while lifting your heels off the ground. See illustration 4.

4、呼气时，两臂由体侧下落至预备姿势。（图5, 6）
5—8同1—4动作，练习次数2—4个八拍。

第二个八拍的最后一拍，两臂由体侧下落交叉于胸前（左手在里，右手在外），同时左脚稍向左开步。（图7—8）

要求：双手用力上托时两臂伸直与身体垂直，同时进行深吸气。

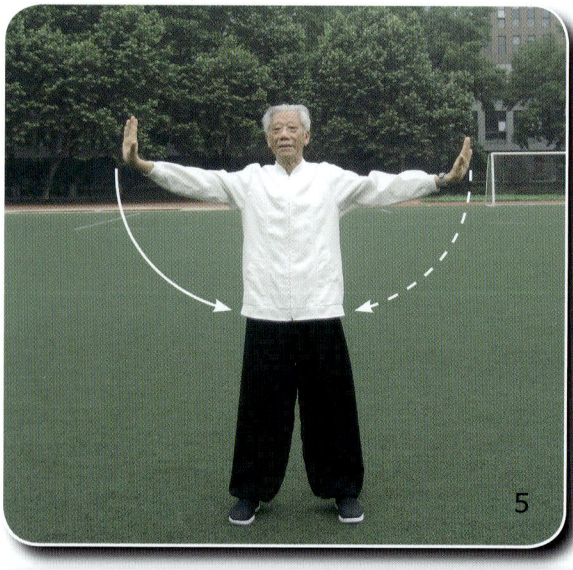
5

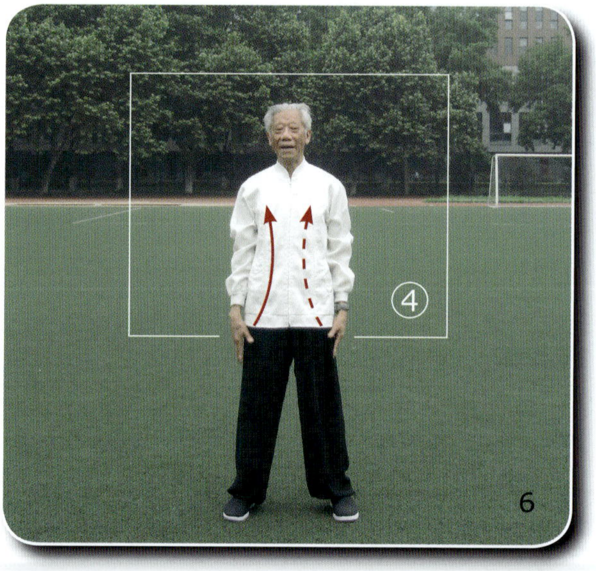

6

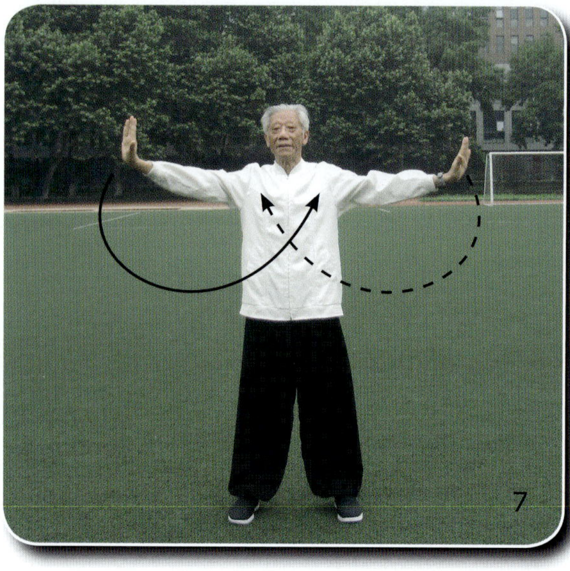
7

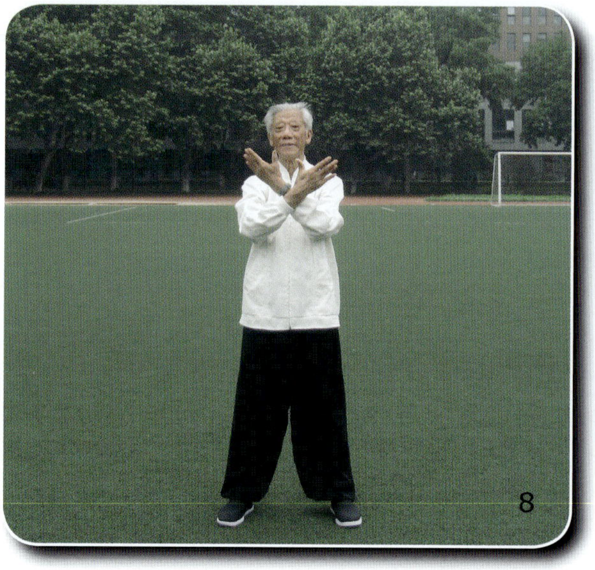
8

4. Mit der Ausatmung werden die Hände bogenförmig zurück in die Ausgangsstellung gebracht. Siehe Bilder 5 und 6.
5. — 8. Die gleichen Bewegungen 1 — 4 werden wiederholt.
Die Bewegungen 1 — 8 zweimal oder viermal ausführen.

Am Ende der Übung die Hände vor der Brust kreuzen. Dabei darauf achten, dass die Hände einen rechten Winkel bilden. Die linke Hand ist dabei innen und die Handflächen sind zur Brust gerichtet. Dabei gleichzeitig den linken Fuß leicht nach links öffnen. Siehe Bilder 7 und 8.

Anforderungen: Die Hände kräftig nach oben strecken, dabei tief einatmen und darauf achten, dass die Arme gerade gestreckt sind und mit dem Körper eine senkrechte Linie bilden.

4. While breathing out guide your hands back to the initial position in a bow. See illustrations 5 and 6.
5. — 8. The same movements 1 — 4 are repeated.
Carry out the movements 1 — 8 two or four times.

At the end of the exercise cross your hands in front of your chest. In doing so mind that your hands form a rectangle. Now your left hand is next to your body and your palms are directed towards your chest. At the same time open your left foot slightly to the left. See illustrations 7 and 8.

Requirements: Stretch your hands upwards powerfully while breathing in deeply and mind that your arms are stretched totally straight and form a vertical line with your body.

## 第二段　拉弓似射雕

预备姿势：两脚平行开立（稍宽于肩），两手自然交叉于胸前（十字手状，左手在里，右手在外）眼看前方。（图1）

动作：

1、吸气时：左手成八字掌向左推出，手臂伸直，掌心向外，食指朝上，右手握拳屈肘于胸前，拳心向里，成拉弓状，同时两腿下蹲成马步，头向左转，眼看左手食指。（图2）

2、呼气时：两腿伸直，头颈转正，同时左手下落与右手在胸前互绕一圈。（图3）

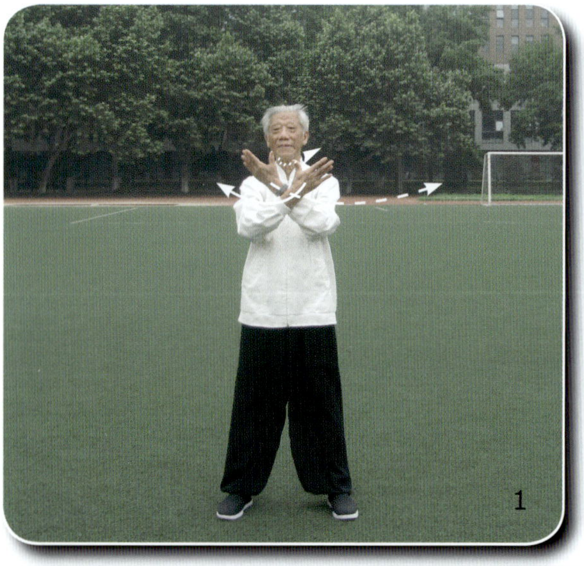
1

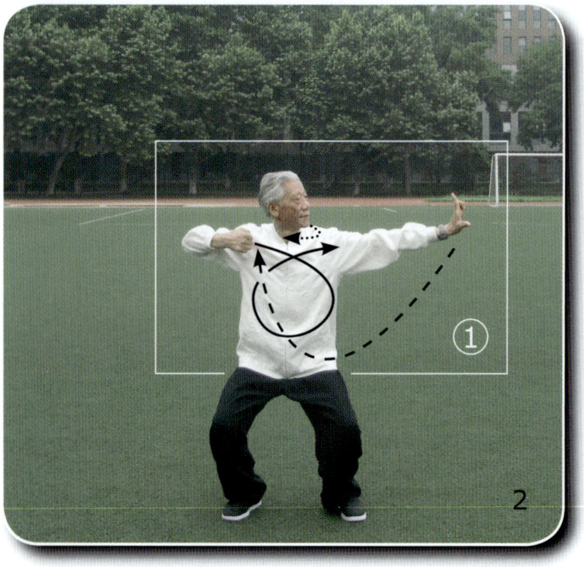

2

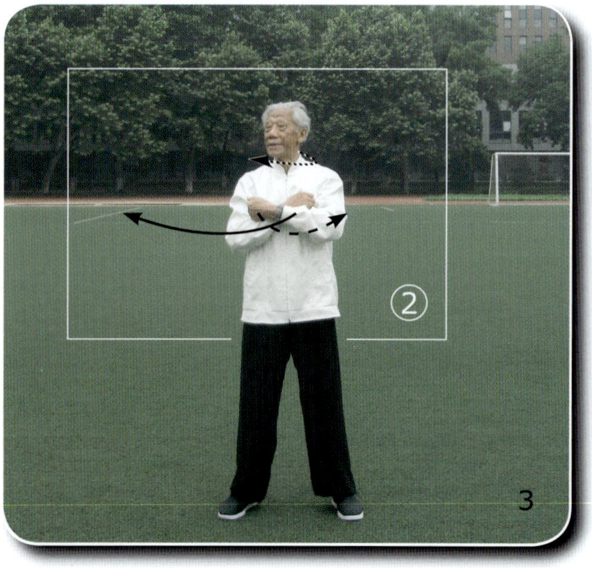

3

## II. Den Bogen spannen und auf den Geier zielen

Ausgangsstellung
Die Füße parallel stellen, etwas breiter als die Schultern. Die Hände vor der Brust kreuzen. Dabei darauf achten, dass die Hände einen rechten Winkel bilden. Die linke Hand ist dabei innen und die Handflächen sind zur Brust gerichtet. Den Blick nach vorne richten. Siehe Bild 1.

1. Mit der Einatmung den linken Arm nach links gerade strecken, die Handfläche schaut nach außen. Die Hand macht dabei das chinesische Zeichen für die Acht (BaZi), d. h. der Daumen wird vom gestreckten Zeigefinger rechtwinklig abgespreizt. Die restlichen Finger werden am zweiten Fingerglied eingerollt. Die rechte Hand zur Faust schließen und vor der Brust nach rechts ziehen, um den Bogen zu spannen. Faust und Ellbogen befinden sich am Ende der Bewegung auf einer Linie. Gleichzeitig die Knie beugen zur Stellung des Pferdes (MaBu). Dabei den Kopf nach links drehen und den Blick auf den linken Zeigefinger richten. Siehe Bild 2.
2. Mit der Ausatmung die Beine strecken, den Kopf nach vorne drehen. Dabei die linke Hand nach unten führen und die Handposition (BaZi) lösen. Die rechte Hand zur Körpermitte führen und die Faust lösen. Anschließend die linke Hand vor der Körpermitte nach oben führen. Nun kreisen beide Hände einmal umeinander. Am Ende sind die Hände wieder vor der Brust gekreuzt. Die rechte Hand ist jetzt innen und die Handflächen schauen zur Brust. Siehe Bild 3.

## II. Drawing the Bow and Aiming at the Vulture

Initial Position
Set your feet parallel, somewhat further apart than your shoulders. Cross your hands in front of your chest. In doing so mind that your hands form a rectangle. Your left hand is next to your body, and your palms are directed towards your chest. Direct your gaze ahead of you. See ill. 1.

1. In breathing in stretch your left arm straight to the left hand side, your palm showing outwards. In doing so your hand forms the Chinese sign for eight (BaZi) which means spreading your thumb off your forefinger in a right angle. Roll in your other fingers at your second knucklejoint. Close your right hand into a fist, drawing it to the right hand side in front of your breast to draw the bow. Your fist and elbow form one line at the end of the movement. At the same time form the Position of the Horse (MaBu) with your legs. In doing so turn your head to the left hand side and direct your gaze towards your left forefinger. See illustration 2.
2. While breathing out stretch your legs again and turn your head to the front. In doing so guide your left hand down and loosen your hand position (BaZi). Next guide your right hand towards the middle of your body and undo your fist. After this guide your left hand upwards in front of the middle of your body. Now both your hands circle once around each other. In the end your hands are crossed once more in front of your chest. Your right hand is next to your body now and your palms show towards your chest. See illustration 3.

3—4同1—2动作，唯有方向相反，（图4，5）练习次数，2—4个八拍，第二个八拍的最后一拍，两脚原地不动，双手合掌于胸前，手指朝上。（图6，7）

要求：拉弓时应两臂争力扩胸，并充分吸气，上体保持中正，马步时两膝垂对足尖。

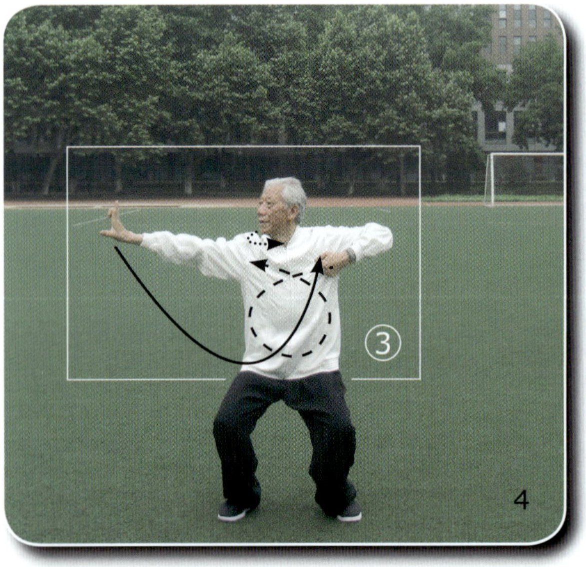
4

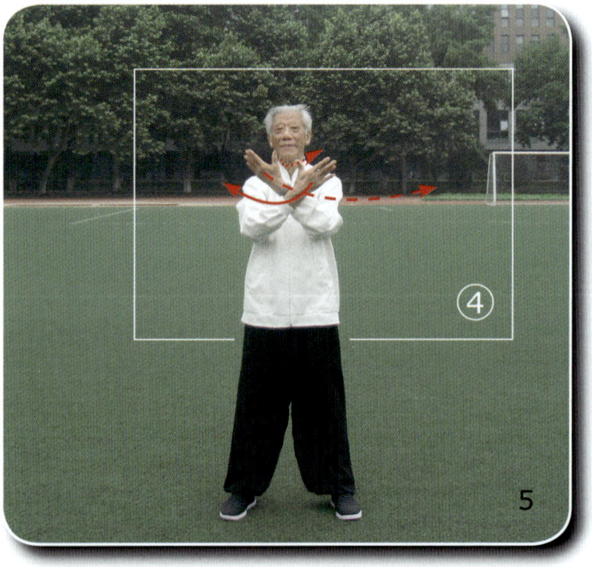
5

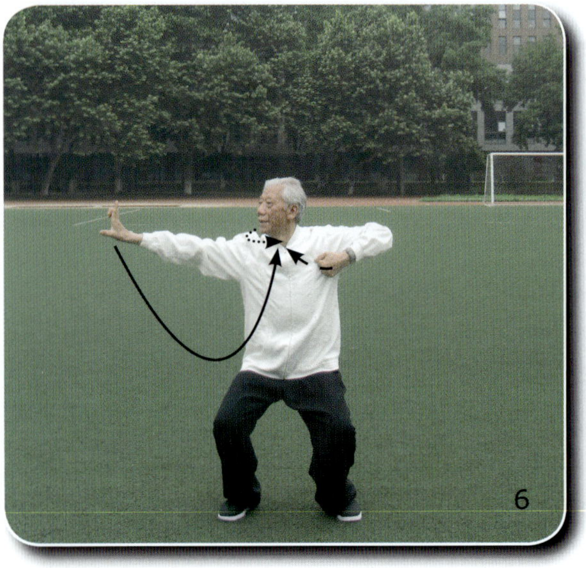
6

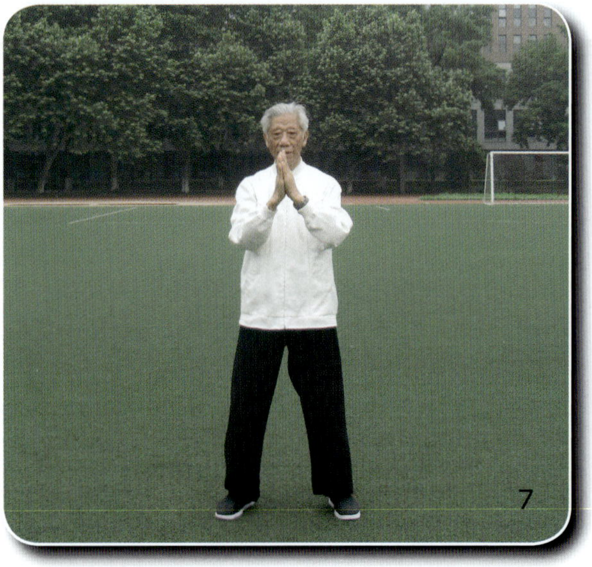
7

3. — 4. Die gleichen Bewegungen wie 1 — 2 in die entgegengesetzte Richtung ausführen. Siehe Bilder 4 und 5.
5. — 8. Die gleichen Bewegungen 1 — 4 werden wiederholt.
Die Bewegungen 1 — 8 zweimal oder viermal ausführen.

Am Ende der Übung die Hände vor der Brust zusammenlegen, die Finger zeigen nach oben. Die Stellung der Füße beibehalten. Siehe Bilder 6 und 7.

Anforderungen: Beim Spannen des Bogens soll die Muskulatur der Arme unter Spannung stehen. Dabei wird die Brust herausgestreckt und es wird vollständig eingeatmet. Der Oberkörper bleibt in einer aufrechten Position. Bei der Stellung des MaBu müssen die Knie in einer Linie mit den Fußspitzen stehen.

3. — 4. Carry out the same movements as 1 — 2 in the opposite direction. See illustrations 4 and 5.
5. — 8. The same movements 1 — 4 are repeated.
Carry out the movements 1 — 8 two or four times.

At the end of the exercises put your hands together in front of your chest, your fingers pointing upwards. Keep the position of your feet. See illustrations 6 and 7.

Requirements: When drawing the bow the muscular system of your arms is meant to be tense. In doing so you project your chest and you breathe in completely. Your upper body remains in an upright postion. In the Position of MaBu your knees must be in one line with your toetips.

## 第三段　单举健脾胃

预备姿势：两脚自然开立，两掌合手于胸前。（图1）

动作：

1、吸气时，两掌根边压边旋转成右掌在上，左掌在下，两腕相靠，接着右手翻掌上托，左手翻掌下按，使两掌上下争力，重心移至右腿，左脚尖点地成左虚步，同时身体向左转体90° 眼看左前方。（图2）

2、呼气时，身体右转，还原成预备姿势，同时两掌重叠于胸前，右手在上，左手在下，两腕相接。（图3）

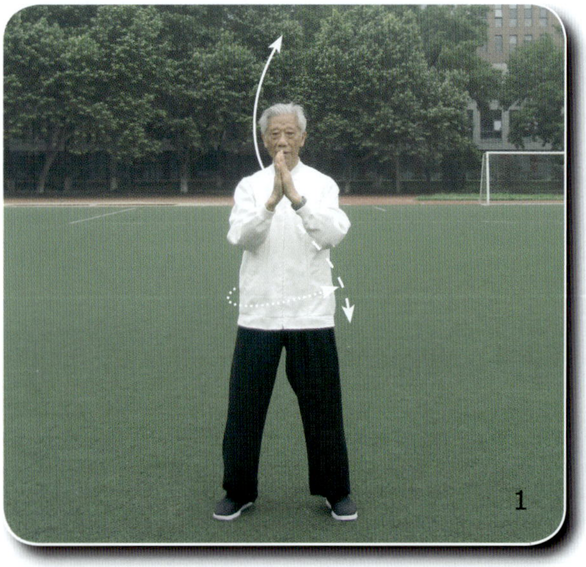

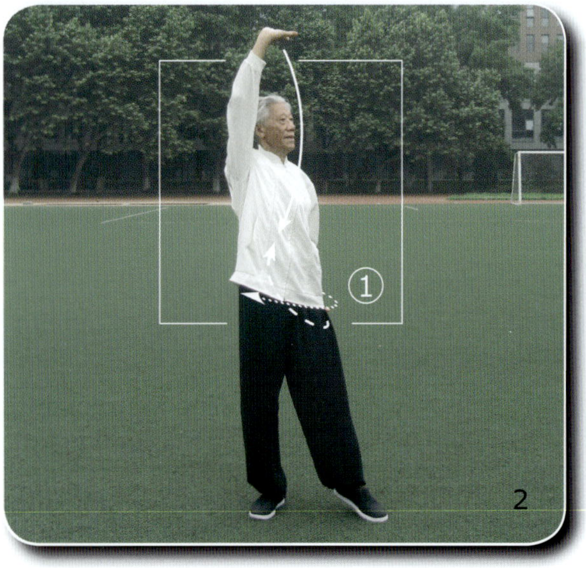


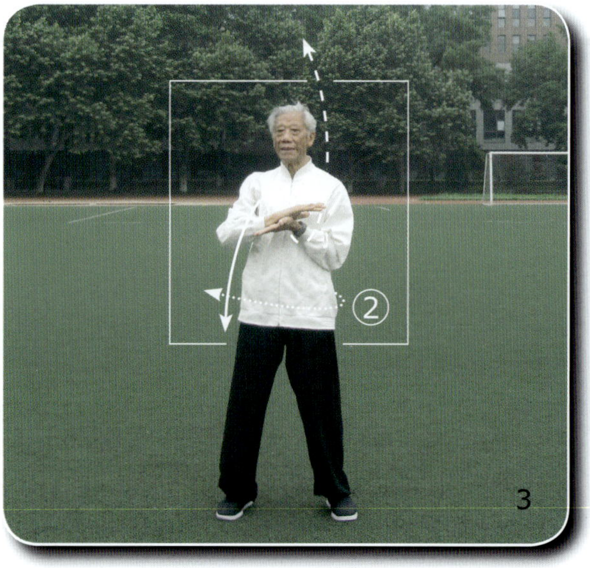

## III. Die Arme einzeln hochheben, um Magen und Milz zu regulieren

Ausgangsstellung
Die Füße auseinander stellen. Die Handflächen vor der Brust zusammenlegen. Siehe Bild 1.

1. Mit der Einatmung die Hände - an den Handgelenken aneinander gedrückt - drehen, so dass die rechte Hand oben und die linke Hand unten ist. Anschließend die rechte Handfläche umdrehen und nach oben über den Kopf strecken, die linke Handfläche umdrehen und nach unten drücken. Beide Hände in entgegengesetzter Richtung anspannen. Gleichzeitig den Schwerpunkt auf das rechte Bein verlagern und den Körper um 90° nach links drehen. Die linke Ferse dabei vom Boden lösen, so dass die Körperdrehung auf den Zehen erfolgen kann. Am Ende der Bewegung befindet man sich in der Stellung des Leeren Schrittes (XuBu). Der Blick folgt der Bewegung. Siehe Bild 2.
2. Mit der Ausatmung den Körper wieder nach rechts in die Ausgangsposition bringen. Dabei die Hände vor der Brust aufeinander legen. Die Hände berühren sich an den Handgelenken, rechte Hand oben, linke Hand unten. Siehe Bild 3.

## III. Lift Your Arms One by One to Regulate Your Stomach and Your Spleen

Initial Position
Put your feet apart. Put your hands together in front of your chest. See illustration 1.

1. In breathing in turn your hands while pressing your wrists against each other so that your right hand is up above and your left hand down under. After this turn your right palm and stretch it up above your head, turn your left palm and press it downwards. Subject your hands to tension into the opposite direction. At the same time shift your centre of gravity onto your right leg and turn your body to the left by 90°. In doing so take your left heel off the ground so that the turning of your body can be carried out on your toes. At the end of the movement you are in the Position of the Empty Step (XuBu). Your gaze follows your movement. See ill. 2.
2. In breathing out get your body back to the right hand side into the initial position. In doing so put your hands one on top of the other in front of your chest. Your hands touch each other at your wrists, your right hand up above, your left hand down under. See illustration 3.

3—4同1—2动作，唯有方向相反。（图4，5）

练习次数:
2—4个八拍，第二个八拍的最后一拍，左臂由左侧下落于体侧，左足向右足靠拢。（图6，7）

要求：两手上下争力与转体同时进行，并配合深吸气，上下肢协调一致。

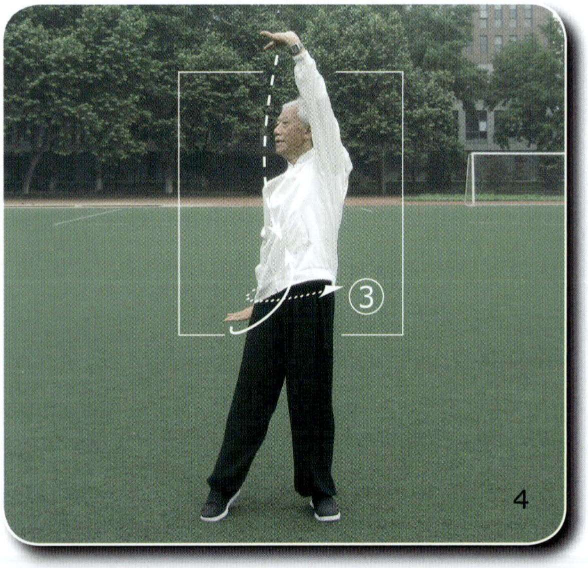

4

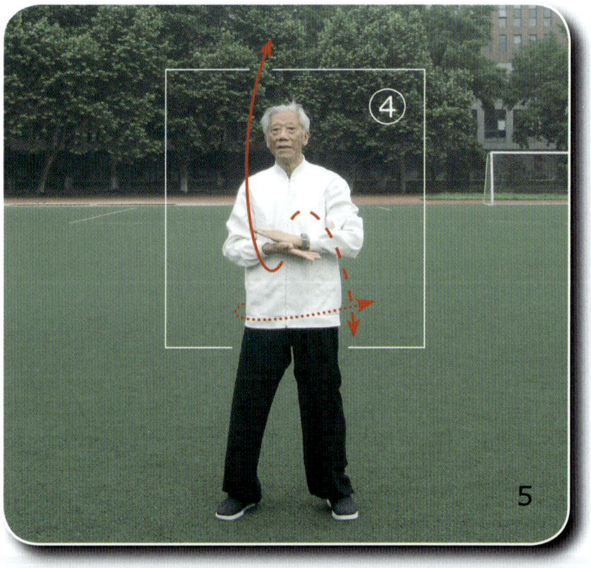

5

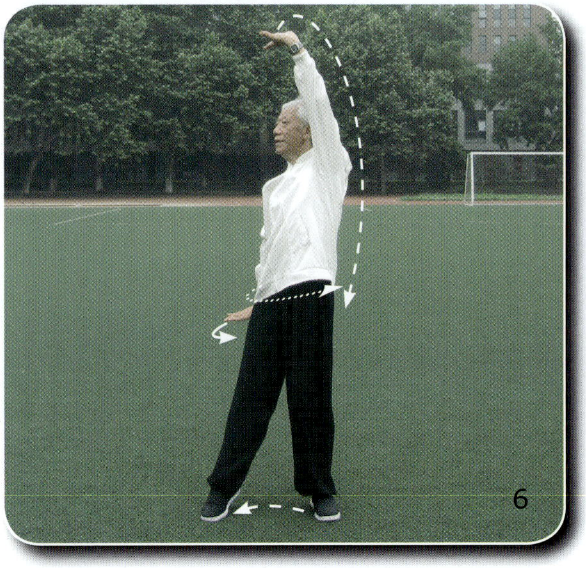
6

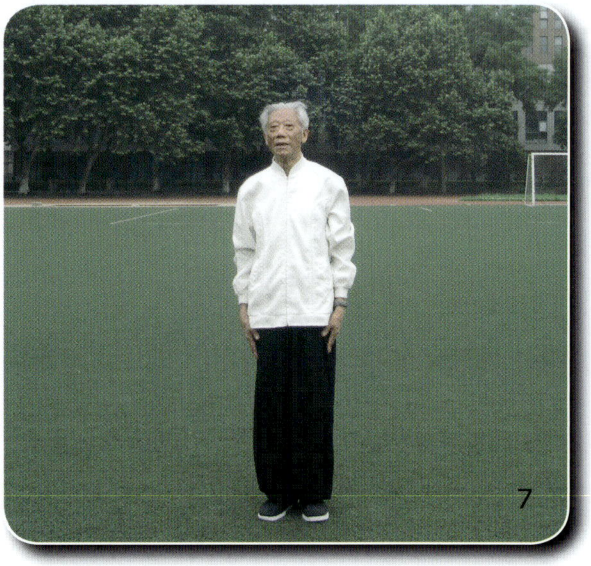
7

3. — 4. Die gleichen Bewegungen wie 1 — 2 in die entgegengesetzte Richtung ausführen. Siehe Bilder 4 und 5.
5. — 8. Die gleichen Bewegungen 1 — 4 werden wiederholt.
Die Bewegungen 1 — 8 zweimal oder viermal ausführen.

Am Ende der Übung den linken Arm nach unten zur linken Körperseite führen. Den linken Fuß an den rechten heransetzen. Siehe Bilder 6 und 7.

Anforderungen: Bei der Körperdrehung gleichzeitig die Hände nach oben und unten anspannen. Dabei tief einatmen und die Bewegungen des Ober- und Unterkörpers aufeinander abstimmen.

3. — 4. Carry out the same movements as 1 — 2 in the opposite direction. See illustrations 4 and 5.
5. — 8. The same movements 1 — 4 are repeated.
Carry out the movements 1 — 8 two or four times.

At the end of the exercise guide your left arm downwards to the left hand side of your body. Put your left foot next to your right foot. See illustrations 6 and 7.

Requirements: During the turning of your body subject your hands to tension upwards and downwards at the same time. In doing so breathe in deeply and synchronize the movements of the upper and lower part of your body.

## 第四段 劳伤向后瞧

预备姿势：两足并立，两臂垂于体侧。（图1）

动作

1、吸气时，左脚向左侧开一步，同时两臂提至侧平举，手心向下（图2）。接着向左转体90°，重心移至左脚，右脚跟提起，两腿伸直，眼看前方。（图3）

2、呼气时，右手下摆向右弧形绕一圈，成屈肘于头前上方，掌心向前，掌指向左，同时左手顺势上摆绕一圈成直臂后勾手，身体向右转体90°，右足向后插步，成歇步下蹲，眼看左勾手。（图4）

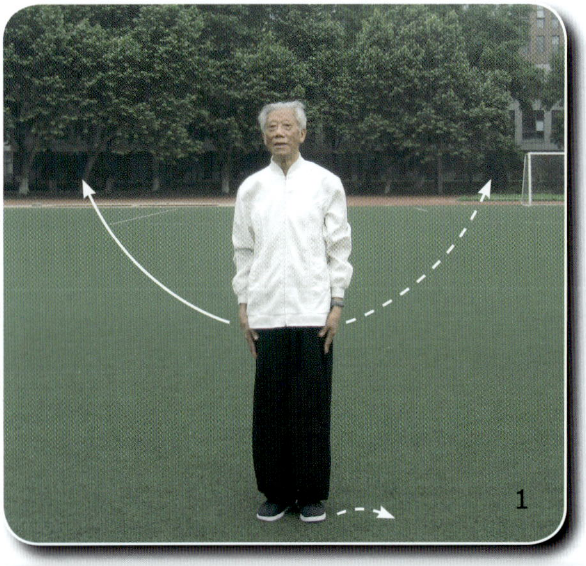


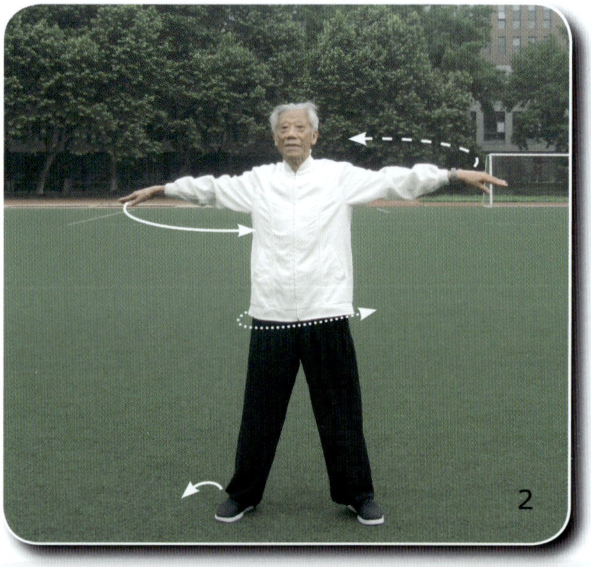


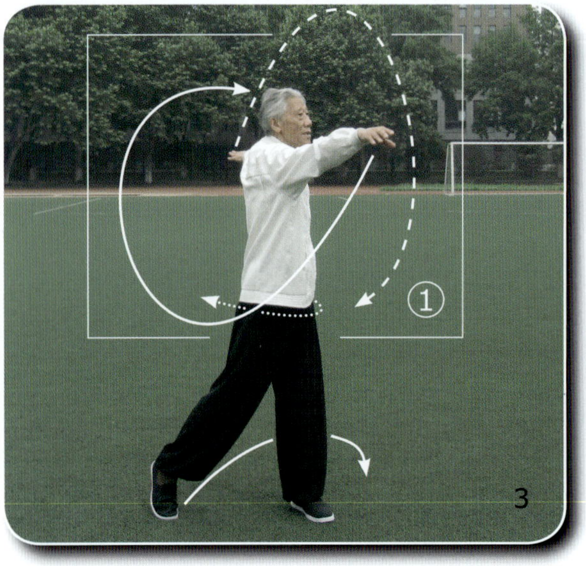


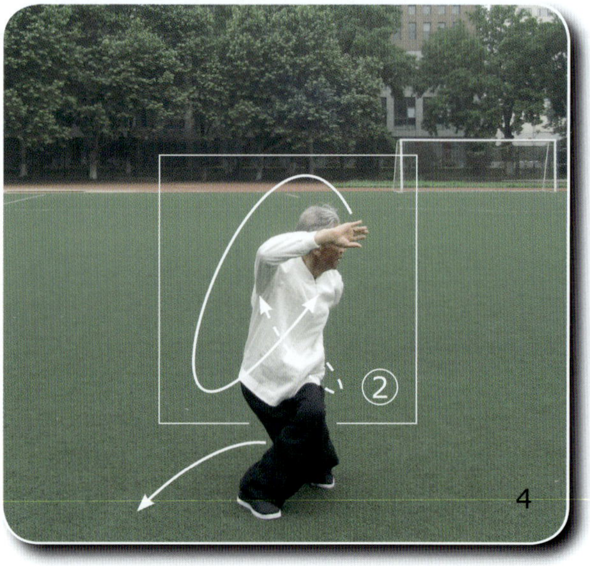

## IV. Die von den Fünf Anstrengungen und Sieben Betrübnissen verursachten Krankheiten vertreiben

Ausgangsstellung

Die Füße nebeneinander stellen. Die Arme hängen an den Seiten des Körpers. Siehe Bild 1.

1. Bei der Einatmung mit dem linken Fuß einen Schritt nach links machen. Dabei die Arme seitlich nach oben bis auf Schulterhöhe anheben, die Handflächen schauen dabei nach unten. Siehe Bild 2. Anschließend den Körper um 90° nach links drehen, den Schwerpunkt auf den linken Fuß verlagern. Die rechte Ferse dabei anheben. Beide Beine sind gestreckt. Siehe Bild 3.
2. Mit der Ausatmung den Körper um 90° nach rechts drehen. Der linke Arm geht dabei nach oben und der rechte Arm nach unten. Die Handflächen schauen dabei nach vorne. Während der linke Arm wieder nach unten geht, steigt der rechte Arm nach oben über den Kopf. Anschließend den rechten Arm im Ellbogen beugen, die Handfläche schaut nach vorne. Beim linken Arm die Finger und den Daumen zur Hakenhand (GouShou) schließen, d. h. die Spitzen des Daumens und der Finger werden zusammengebracht und das Handgelenk nach unten gebeugt. Während der Bewegung der Arme wird der rechte Fuß hinter den linken Fuß gesetzt. Dabei geht man in die Hocke und befindet sich dann in der Stellung des Ruhenden Schrittes (XieBu). Der Blick geht dabei zur linken Hand. Siehe Bild 4.

## IV. Expel the Illnesses Caused by the Five Strains and the Seven Afflictions

Initial Position

Put your feet next to each other. Your arms dangle at the sides of your body. See illustration 1.

1. In breathing in make one step with your left foot towards your left hand side. In doing so lift your arms at your sides upwards to shoulder height, your palms showing downwards while doing so. See ill. 2. Following this turn your body to your left by 90° and shift your point of gravity onto your left foot. In doing so lift your right heel. Both your legs are stretched. See ill. 3.
2. In breathing out turn your body to the right by 90°. In doing so your left arm goes upwards and your right arm downwards. Your palms show ahead of you while you do so. While your left arm goes down again, your right arm is raised up above your head. Following this you bow your right arm at your elbow, your palm showing ahead of you. At your left arm close your fingers and your thumb to Hookhand (GouShou), putting the tips of your thumb and your fingers together and bending your wrist downwards. During the movement of the arms your right foot is put behind your left foot. In doing so you squat into the Position of the Resting Stance (XieBu). In doing so your gaze is directed towards your left hand. See illustration 4.

3、吸气时，身体起立，右脚收回原位，同时两臂弧形绕至胸前交叉，右手在外，掌心均向内。（图5）
4、呼气时，左脚向右脚靠拢，同时两臂向左右翻掌经体侧下落成预备式。（图6, 7）

5—8同1—4动作，唯有方向相反，练习次数2—4个八拍。

要求：歇步下蹲的深度因人而宜，但均需转头后看勾手。

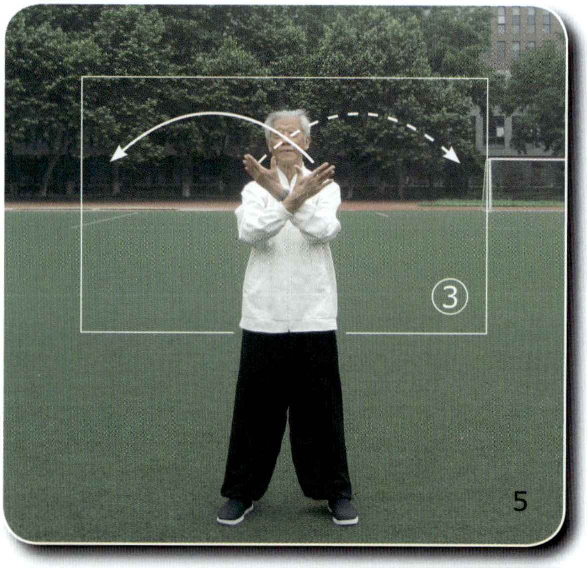


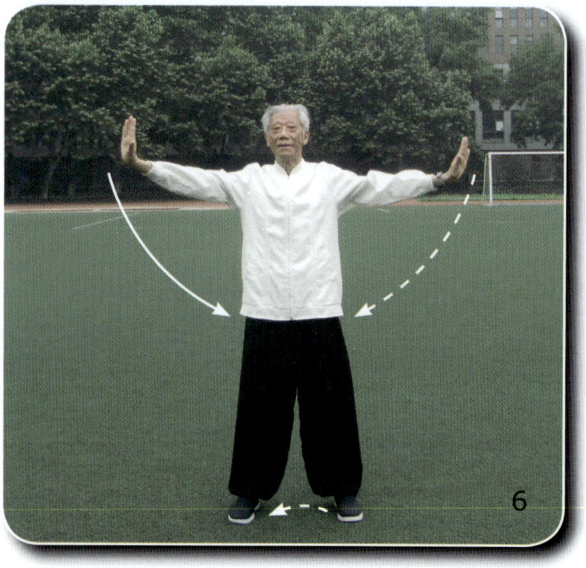


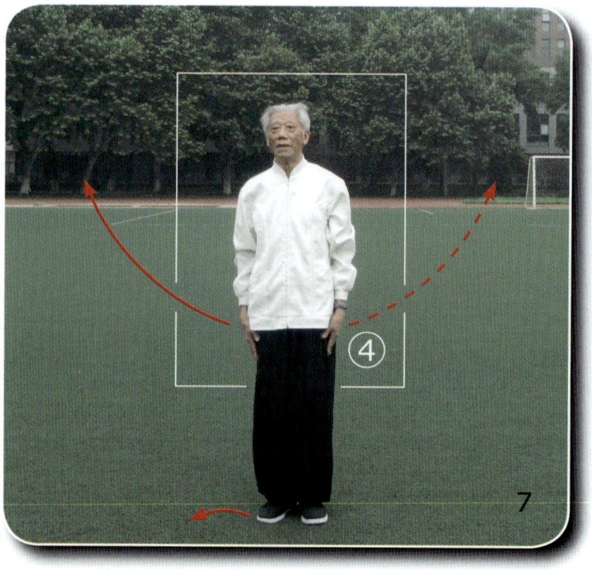

3. Mit der Einatmung wieder aufstehen. Den rechten Fuß zum schulterbreiten Stand zurücksetzen. Gleichzeitig beide Arme vor der Brust kreuzen, der rechte Arm wird über den linken Arm gekreuzt, die Handflächen zeigen zum Körper. Siehe Bild 5.
4. Mit der Ausatmung werden die Arme in einem Bogen zur linken und zur rechten Körperseite in die Ausgangsposition gebracht. Die Handflächen dabei nach außen drehen und gleichzeitig den linken Fuß wieder an den rechten Fuß heransetzen. Siehe Bilder 6 und 7.

5. — 8. Die gleichen Bewegungen 1 — 4 werden in die entgegensetzte Richtung wiederholt. Die Bewegungen 1 — 8 zweimal oder viermal ausführen.

Anforderungen: Die Tiefe der Position des Ruhenden Schrittes (XieBu) soll individuell gestaltet sein. Wichtig ist, dass der Blick zur Hakenhand (GouShou) geht.

3. In breathing in you get up again. You put back your right foot to shoulder breadth stance. At the same time cross both your arms in front of your chest, crossing your right arm over your left arm, your palms showing to your body. See illustration 5.
4. In breathing out you guide your arms in a bow to the left and the right hand side of your body to the initial position. In doing so your palms are turned outwards, and at the same time you set your left foot back next to your right foot. See illustrations 6 and 7.

5. — 8. The same movements 1 — 4 are repeated into the opposite direction.
Carry out the movements 1 — 8 two or four times.

Requirements: The lowness of the Position of the Resting Stance (XieBu) shall be formed individually. It is important that your gaze goes towards your hookhand (GouShou).

## 第五段　摇摆去心火

预备姿势：两脚并立，两手垂于体侧。（图1）

动作

1、左脚向左侧开一步（略宽于肩），同时两手侧平举（手心向下）（图2），接着身体向左屈体，用右手拍击左腿足三里，左手随体转向后直臂摆出，同时左足尖上跷（左腿伸直）右腿屈膝，头向左摆，体重落在右腿上。（图3）

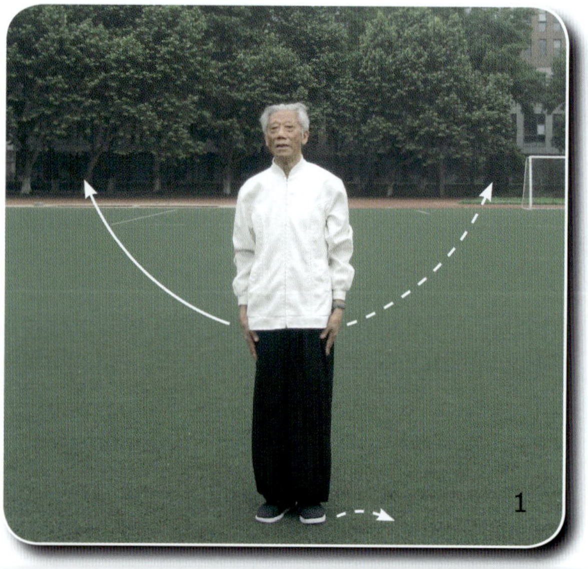


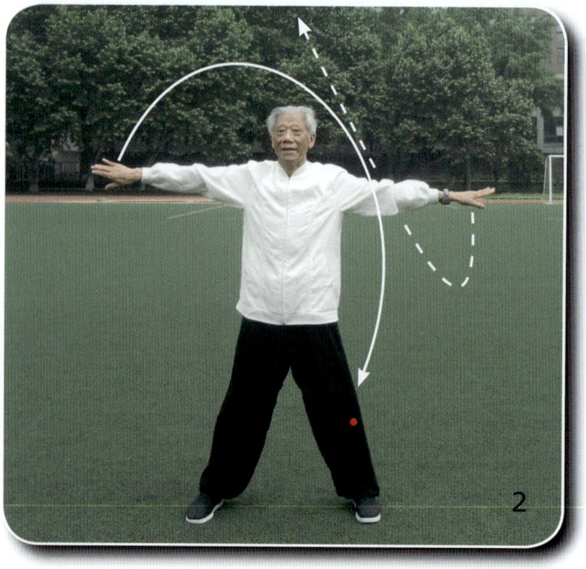


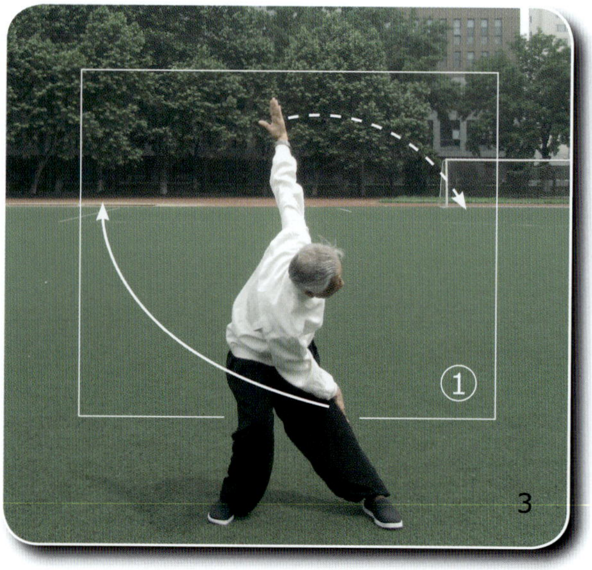

## V. Mit Wiegen und Wedeln die innere Hitze aus dem Herzen vertreiben

Ausgangsstellung
Die Füße nebeneinander stellen. Die Arme hängen an den Seiten herab. Siehe Bild 1.

1. Mit dem linken Fuß einen Schritt nach links machen (etwas breiter als die Schultern). Die Hände dabei bis zur Höhe der Schultern anheben (Handflächen nach unten). Siehe Bild 2. Anschließend den Oberkörper nach links vorne bücken und dabei das rechte Bein beugen. Den Schwerpunkt dabei auf das rechte Bein verlagern und die Fußspitze des linken Fußes vom Boden lösen (das linke Bein bleibt dabei gerade). Der Kopf folgt dabei der Bewegung nach links, während man mit der rechten Hand auf die Außenseite des Beines etwas unterhalb des linken Knies schlägt, auf den Punkt ZuSanLi (Drei Meilen am Bein) des Magenmeridians. Die linke Hand geht dabei weiter nach hinten und oben. Siehe Bild 3.

## V. Expel the Inner Heat from Your Heart by Rocking and Wagging

Initial Position
Put your feet next to each other. Your arms dangle at your sides. See illustration 1.

1. Make one step to the left with your left foot (somewhat broader than your shoulders). In doing so lift your hands up to shoulder height (palms downwards). See illustration 2. Following this bow the upper part of your body downwards to your left hand front side and at the same time bend your right leg. In doing so shift your centre of gravity onto your right leg and take the tip of your left foot off the ground (in keeping your left leg straight). Your head follows the movement to the left hand side while with your right hand you slap at the outward side of your leg somewhat beneath your left knee onto the Point ZuSanLi (Three Miles on the Leg) of the Meridian of the Stomach. While doing so your left hand goes further back and upwards. See illustration 3.

2、上体转正，两脚原地不动，双臂经侧平举，向右做动作（动作与1相同，方向相反）。（图4，5）

3、身体转正，两臂经体侧向前向上向后摆出，使两臂屈肘，两手拍击大椎穴，同时两腿成马步。（图6，7）

4、两腿伸直，两臂向前直臂落于体侧，同时两手握拳，中指扣劳宫穴。（图8）

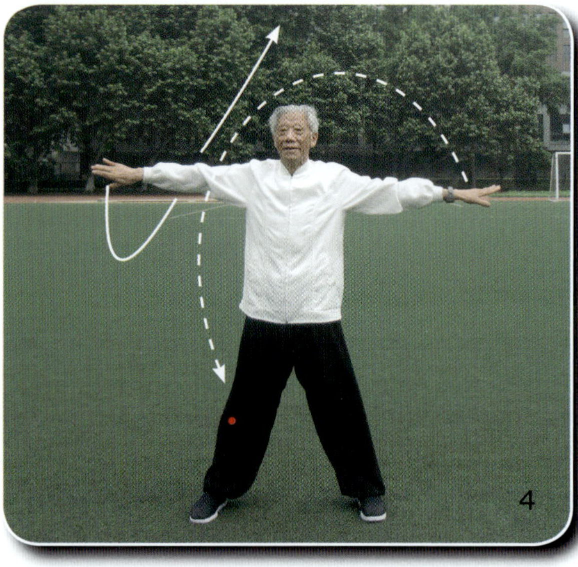
4

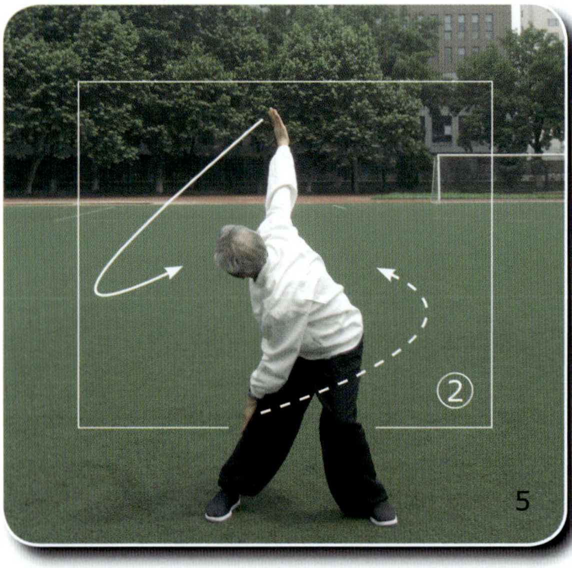

5

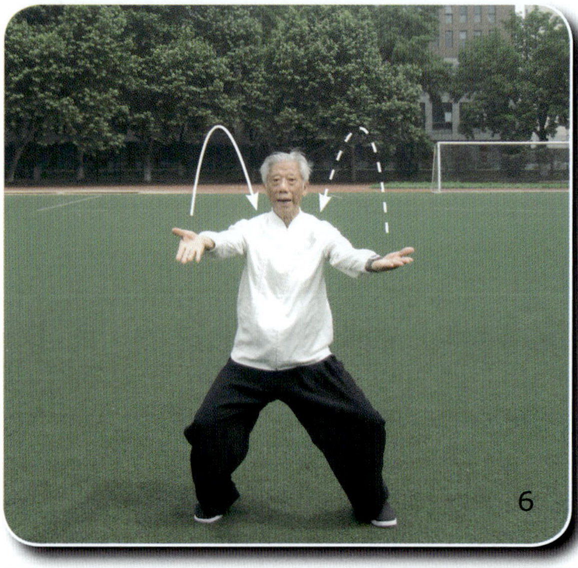
6

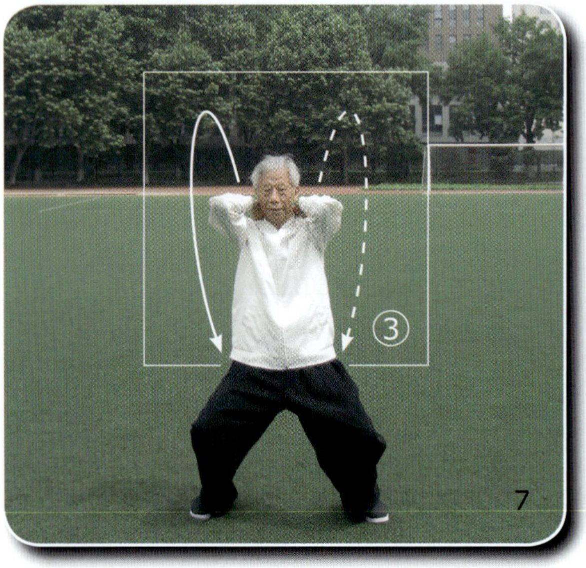

7

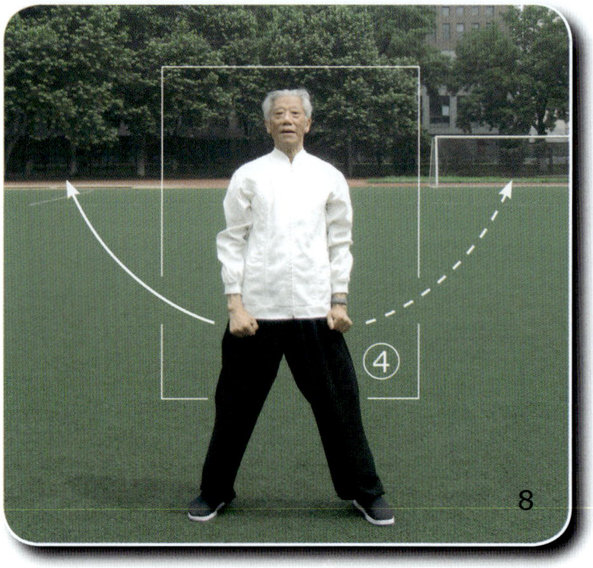

8

2. Den Oberkörper aufrichten und die Hände wieder bis auf Schulterhöhe bringen (Handflächen nach unten). Die Füße bleiben an der Position stehen. Anschließend den Oberkörper nach rechts vorne bücken und dabei das linke Bein beugen. Den Schwerpunkt dabei auf das linke Bein verlagern und die Fußspitze des rechten Fußes vom Boden lösen. (Das rechte Bein bleibt dabei gerade). Der Kopf folgt dabei der Bewegung nach rechts, während man mit der linken Hand auf die Außenseite des Beines etwas unterhalb des rechten Knies auf den Punkt ZuSanLi schlägt. Die rechte Hand geht dabei weiter nach hinten und oben. Siehe Bilder 4 und 5.
3. Den Körper nach vorne drehen und in eine aufrechte Position bringen. Beide Arme entlang des Körpers nach vorne oben bewegen, die Ellenbogen beugen, mit den Händen auf die Schulterblätter zum Punkt DaZhui (Großer Wirbel) des Lenkergefäßes schlagen. Man befindet sich nun in der Stellung des Pferdes (MaBu). Siehe Bilder 6 und 7.
4. Die Beine wieder strecken und die Arme gestreckt (Handflächen nach vorne) nach unten führen. Dabei die Hände zur Faust schließen und mit dem jeweiligen Mittelfinger der Hand den Punkt LaoGong (Im Zentrum der Arbeit) des Perikardmeridians drücken. Siehe Bild 8.

2. Straighten your upper body and guide your hands up to shoulder height again (your palms downwards). Your feet remain in the very position. Following this bow the upper part of your body towards the front right hand side and at the same time bow your left leg. In doing so shift your centre of gravity onto your left leg and take the tip of your right foot off the ground. (In doing so your right leg keeps straight). During this procedure your head swings to the right hand side while with your left hand you slap at the outside of your leg somewhat beneath your right knee onto ZuSanLi Point. In doing so your right hand goes further back and up. See illustrations 4 and 5.
3. Turn your body to the front and get it into an upright position. Move both your arms alongside your body to the front and upwards, bow your elbows, slap with your hands onto your shoulder-blades towards DaZhui Point (Big Vertebra) of the Leader Vessel. Now you are in the Position of the Horse (MaBu). See illustrations 6 and 7.
4. Straighten your legs again and guide your arms downwards in a straightened fashion (palms to the front). In doing so close your hands into a fist and with the respective middle finger of each hand press LaoGong Point (In the Centre of Work) of the Pericardial Meridian. See illustration 8.

5—8重复1—4动作，唯有第5动不用出左脚，第8动左脚向右脚靠拢。（图9—15）

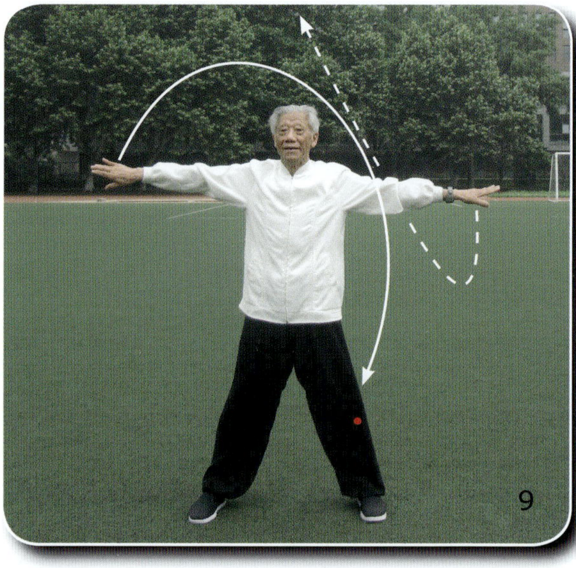
9

练习次数：2—4个八拍，第二个八拍和第一个八拍动作相同，其方向相反，到最后一拍时，右足向左足靠拢，两臂垂直于体侧。（图15）

要求：动作幅度宜大，采用自然呼吸。

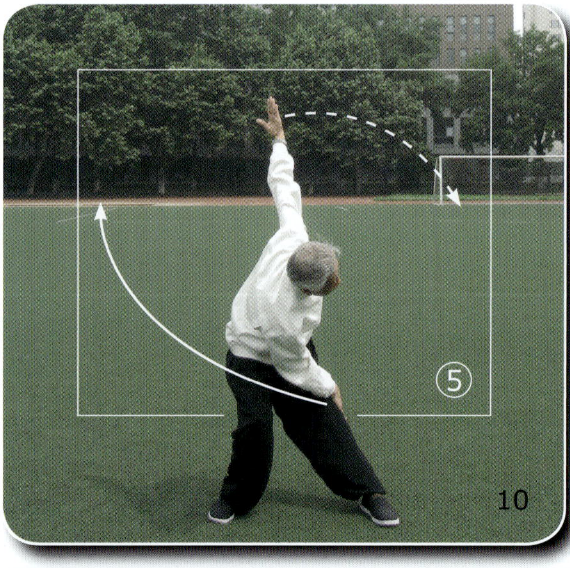

10

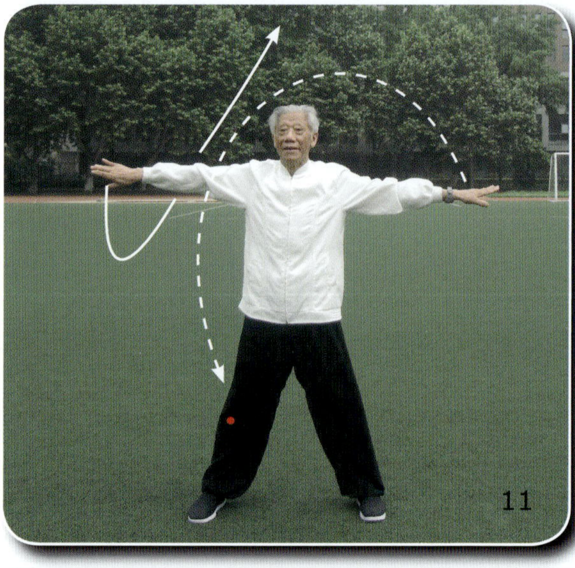
11

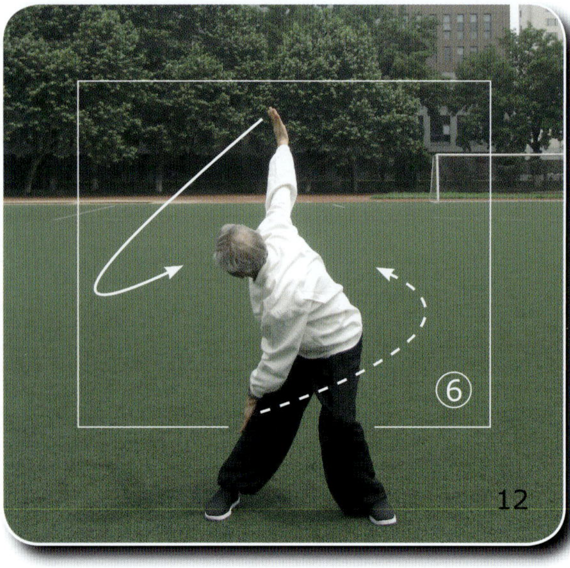

12

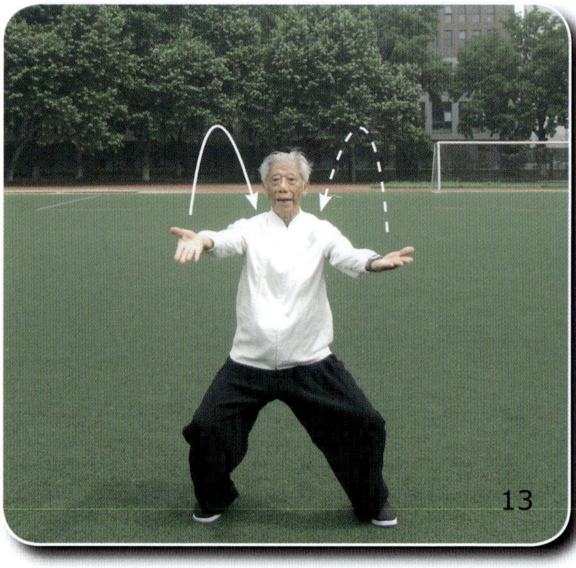
13

5. — 8. Die gleichen Bewegungen 1 — 4 werden wiederholt. Die Position 4 ist die Ausgangsstellung für die Position 5 (d.h. die Position der Füße wird nicht verändert). Am Ende der Übung wird der linke Fuß zum rechten Fuß zurückgebracht. Siehe Bilder 9 - 15.
Die Bewegungen 1 — 8 zweimal oder viermal ausführen.

Beim zweiten Durchgang die gleichen Bewegungen zur anderen Seite ausführen. Am Ende des zweiten Durchganges den rechten Fuß zum linken Fuß und die Arme zu den Körperseiten zurückbringen. Siehe Bild 15.

Anforderungen: Die Schwingungsweite der Bewegungen soll groß sein. Natürlich atmen bei der Übung.

5. — 8. The same movements as 1 — 4 are repeated. Position 4 is the initial position for position 5 (which means that the position of your feet is not changed). At the end of the exercise the left foot is guided back to the right foot. See illustrations 9 - 15.
Carry out the movements 1 — 8 two or four times.

During the second sequence carry out the same movements into the opposite direction. At the end of the second sequence guide back your right foot to your left foot and your arms to the sides of your body. See illustrations 9 - 15.

Requirements: The amplitude of the movements shall be wide. Breathe naturally during the exercise.

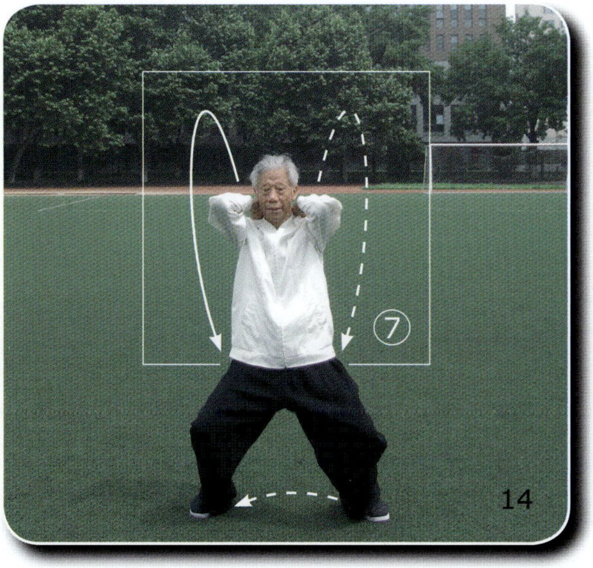

14

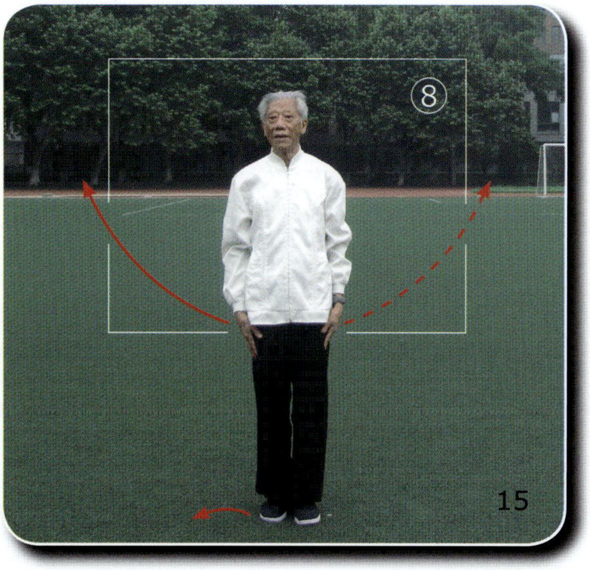

15

## 第六段　躬身固肾腰

预备姿势：两脚并立，双手垂于体侧。（图1）

动作

1、吸气时，两掌由外旋经体侧向后向上摆至头上方直臂合掌（眼看手掌）。（图2）

2、呼气时，两手下落至胸前十指交叉（图3），身体前屈，两腿伸直，双手下按成躬身触地（或足背）。（图4）

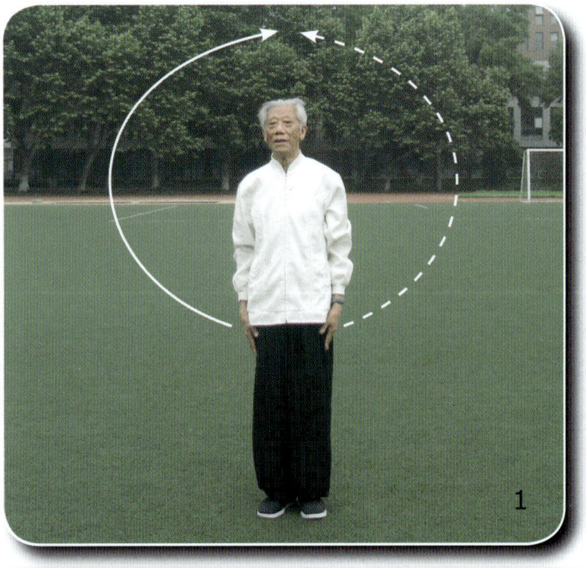


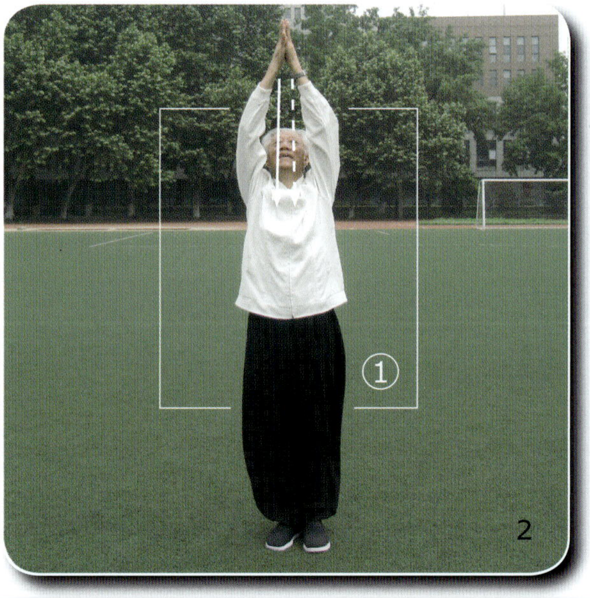


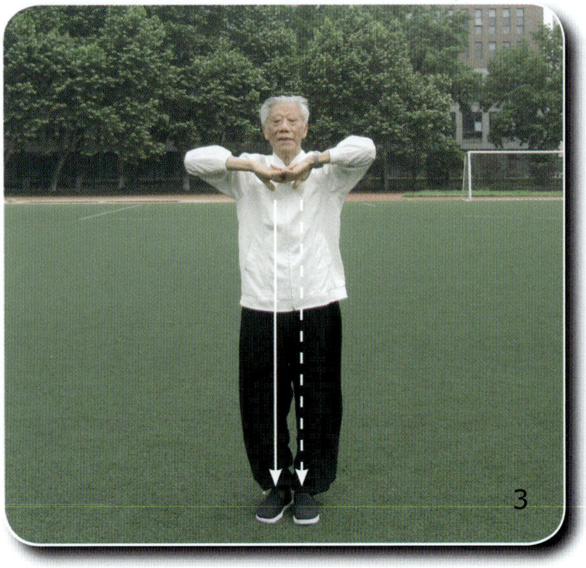


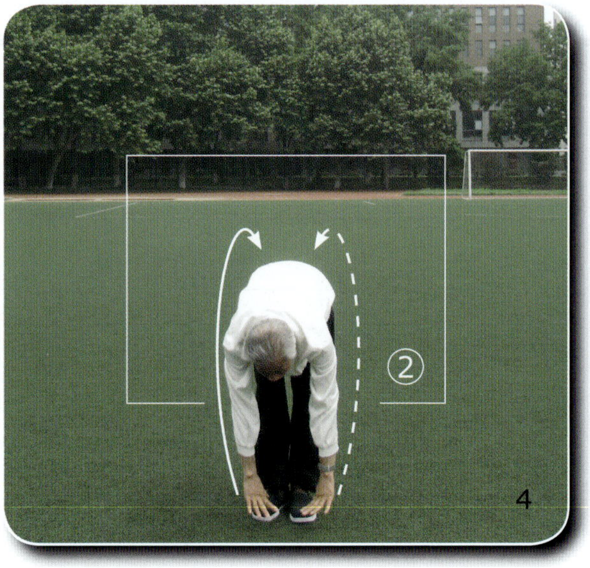

## VI. Tief beugen, um die Nieren und den Hüftbereich zu stärken

Ausgangsstellung
Die Füße nebeneinander stellen. Die Arme hängen an den Seiten des Körpers. Siehe Bild 1.

1. Mit der Einatmung die Hände umdrehen (Handflächen schauen nach außen) und dann die Arme nach oben über den Kopf führen, bis sich die Handflächen berühren. Der Blick geht nach oben zu den Handflächen. Siehe Bild 2.
2. Mit der Ausatmung die Hände nach unten bringen und die Finger dabei vor der Brust kreuzen. Siehe Bild 3. Den Oberkörper nach vorne beugen, die Beine bleiben dabei gestreckt. Die Hände möglichst weit zum Boden führen. Siehe Bild 4.

## VI. Bend Deep Down to Strengthen Your Kidneys and the Region of Your Hips

Initial Position
Put your feet next to each other. Your arms dangle at the sides of your body. See illustration 1.

1. In breathing in turn your hands (your palms showing outwards) and then guide your arms upwards above your head, until your palms touch each other. Your gaze is directed upwards at your palms. See illustration 2.
2. In breathing out guide your hands downwards and cross your fingers in front of your chest in doing so. See illustration 3. Bow the upper part of your body to the front side keeping your legs straight. Guide your hands towards the ground as far as you possibly can. See illustration 4.

3、吸气时，两掌分开，由足背向后经两腿后侧，随上体抬起，两手摩运至肾俞并同时提肛缩肾，双足跟提起。（图5）
4、呼气时，两掌由两肾向下摩运至体侧，同时足跟着地。（图6）

5—8同1—4动作练习次数：2—4个八拍。

要求：躬身下按尽量充分（深度因人而宜），躬身时不低头，两腿不弯曲。第三动吸气时，重在提肛缩肾。第四动呼气时，须松腹松肛。

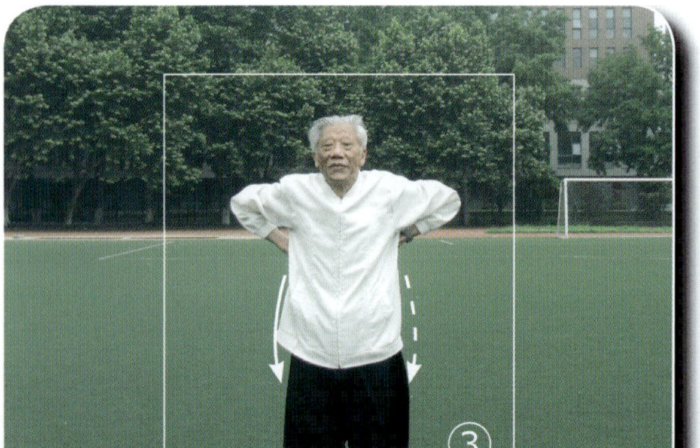


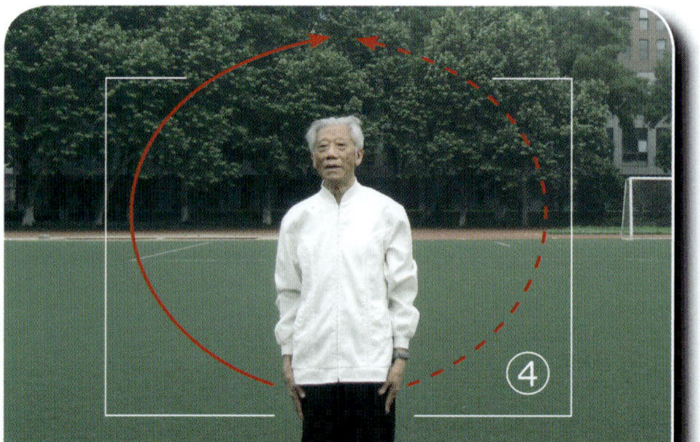

3. Bei der Einatmung die Hände voneinander lösen und beim anschließenden Aufrichten des Oberkörpers mit den Händen über die Fußrücken, dann an der Rückseite der Beine nach oben streifen bis zum Punkt ShenShu (Transportpunkt zu den Nieren) des Blasenmeridians. Die Hände dabei schalenförmig über die Nieren stülpen, gleichzeitig Schließmuskel und Bauch anspannen. Die Fersen vom Boden lösen. Siehe Bild 5.
4. Mit der Ausatmung streifen die Handflächen an den Nieren mit sanftem Druck nach unten bis zu den Außenseiten des Körpers, während man die Fersen wieder zum Boden bringt. Siehe Bild 6.

5. — 8. Die gleichen Bewegungen 1 — 4 werden wiederholt.
Die Bewegungen 1 — 8 zweimal oder viermal ausführen.

Anforderungen: Den Oberkörper so weit wie möglich beugen (jeder so weit er kann). Den Kopf bei der Beugung nach vorne aufrichten und nicht hängen lassen. Der Schwerpunkt bei der dritten Bewegung liegt bei der Anspannung des Schließmuskels und des Bauches während der Einatmung. Bei der vierten Bewegung werden bei der Ausatmung der Schließmuskel und der Bauch wieder entspannt.

3. In breathing in take your hands off each other. While straightening the upper part of your body stroke with your hands along the backs of your feet, then along the back parts of your legs upwards to the Point ShenShu (Point of Transport to the Kidneys) of the Urinary Bladder Channel. In doing so make a cup of your hands putting them over the kidneys, at the same time put your sphincter and your stomach under tension. Take your heels off the ground. See illustration 5.
4. In breathing out your palms stroke downwards along the kidneys with soft pressure right to the sides of your body while you put your heels back to the ground. See illustration 6.

5. — 8. The same movements as 1 — 4 are repeated.
Carry out the movements 1 — 8 two or four times.

Requirements: Bend the upper part of your body as far as possible (everbody as far as he/she possibly can). While you are bending take your head up front and do not keep it bowed. The crucial point in the third movement is in putting your sphincter and your stomach into tension while breathing in. In the fourth movement your sphincter and stomach are relaxed again in breathing out.

## 第七段　瞪目增气力

预备姿势：两足并立，双手垂于体侧。（图1）

动作：

1、左脚向左侧开一步，体重移至左腿，右腿伸直，成左侧弓步，同时右手立掌向右前方直臂挑出，掌心向外，掌指向上，与眼同高，左手握拳收于左腰侧（拳心向上），上体向左转动，右臂随腰转，向左移动，目瞪右掌指。（图2，3）

2、两腿自然伸直，同时右手握拳（手心向上）收于右腰侧。（图4，5）

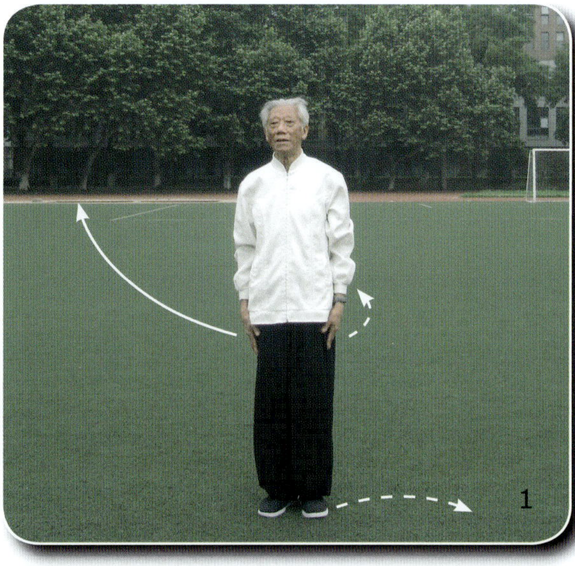
1

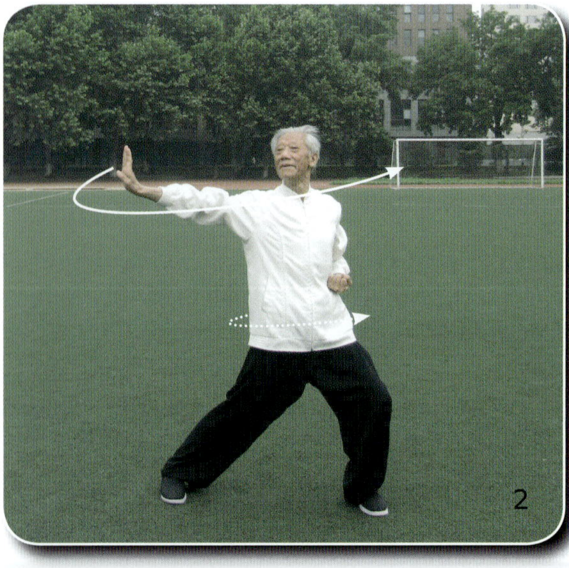
2

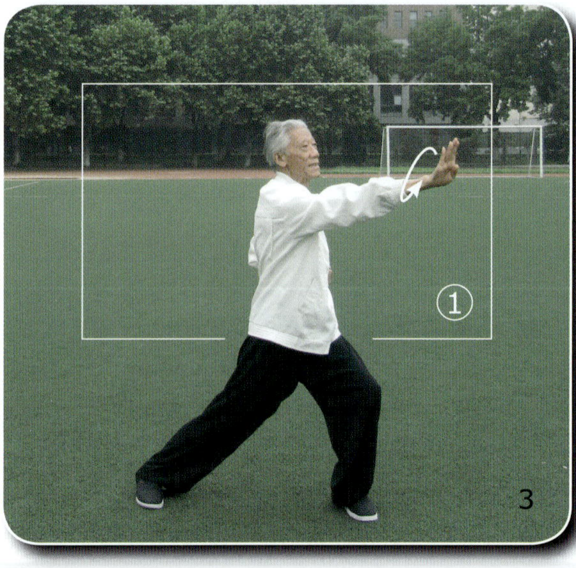
3

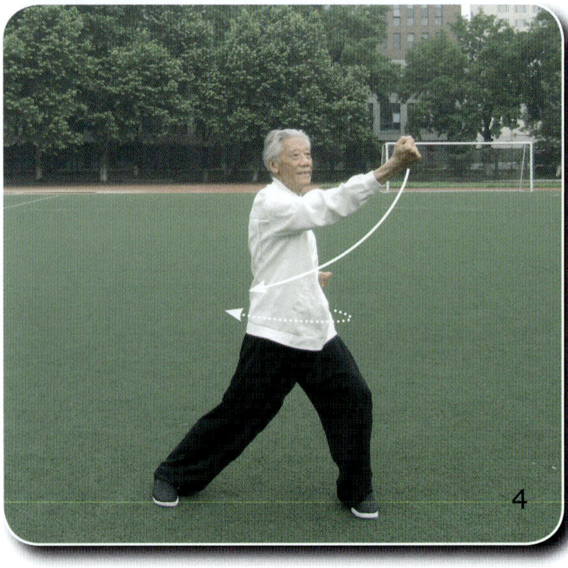
4

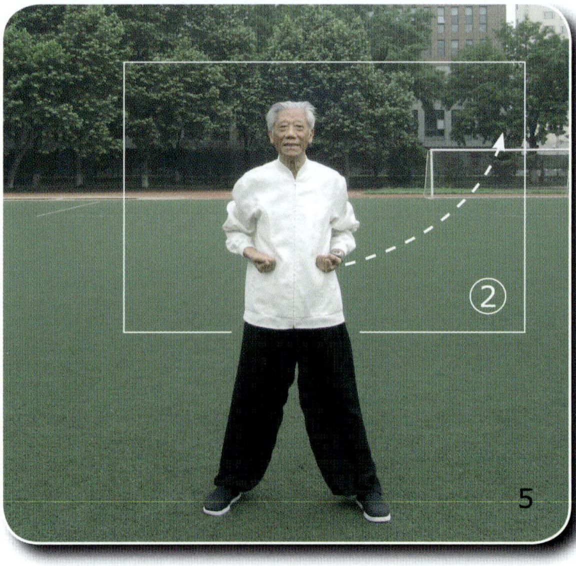
5

## VII. Die Augen weit öffnen – Qi vermehren

Ausgangsstellung
Die Füße parallel stellen. Die Arme hängen an den Seiten des Körpers. Siehe Bild 1.

1. Den linken Fuß einen Schritt nach links bewegen. Den Schwerpunkt auf das linke Bein verlagern, das rechte Bein bleibt gerade bei einem Seitlichen Bogenschritt (GongBu). Gleichzeitig die rechte Hand nach vorne rechts strecken. Der Arm wird dabei gerade gestreckt, Handfläche nach außen, Fingerspitzen nach oben auf Augenhöhe. Die linke Hand umdrehen (Handfläche nach oben), zur Faust schließen und zur Taille bringen. Siehe Bild 2. Den Oberkörper nach links drehen und so den rechten Arm nach links bringen. Der Arm wird dabei nicht bewegt, die Drehung erfolgt nur über die Taille. Mit weit geöffneten Augen zur rechten Hand blicken. Bild 3.
2. Die Beine ganz natürlich strecken. Gleichzeitig die rechte Hand zur Faust schließen (Handfläche nach oben) und zurück zur rechten Seite der Taille ziehen. Siehe Bilder 4 und 5.

## VII. Open Your Eyes Wide – Enhancing Qi

Initial position
Put your feet parallel. Your arms dangle at the sides of your body. See illustration 1.

1. Move your left foot one step to the left hand side. Shift your centre of gravity onto your left leg, your right leg remaining straight in a Lateral Bow Step (GongBu). At the same time stretch your right hand to the front right hand side. In doing so your arm is stretched out, palm outwards, the tips of your fingers at the height of your eyes. Turn your left hand (your palm upwards), close it into a fist and guide it towards your waist. See illustration 2. Turn your upper body to the left and in this way guide your right arm to the left hand side. In carrying this out you do not move your arm, the turning is completed by your waist only. You gaze at your right hand with your eyes wide open. See illustration 3.
2. Stretch your legs quite naturally. At the same time close your right hand into a fist (your palm upwards) and draw it back towards the right hand side of your waist. See illustrations 4 and 5.

3—4与1—2动作相同，唯有方向相反（而右脚无需向右开步）。（图6—9）

练习次数，左右重复做2—4个八拍。

第二个八拍的最后一拍，双手垂于体侧。（图10）

要求：挑掌握拳稍用力，脚趾抓地，瞪目观掌，自然呼吸。

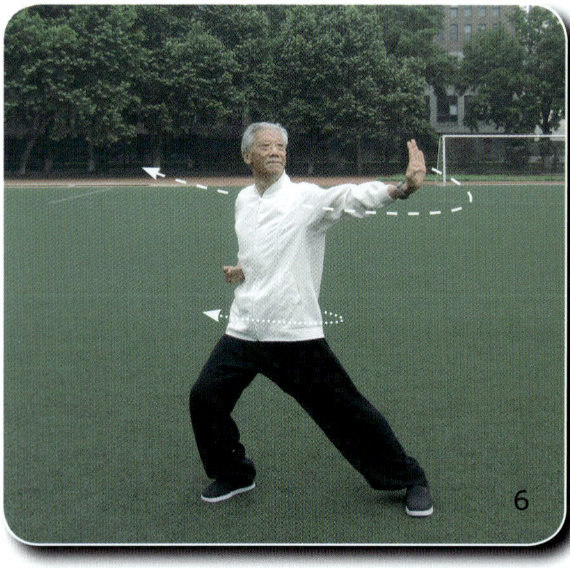
6

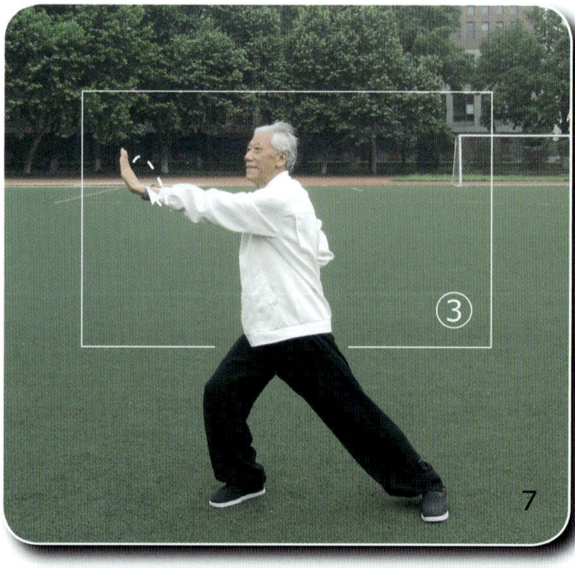

7

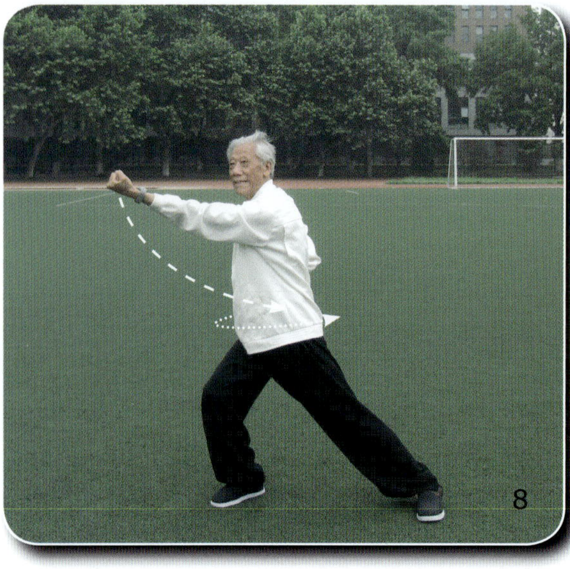
8

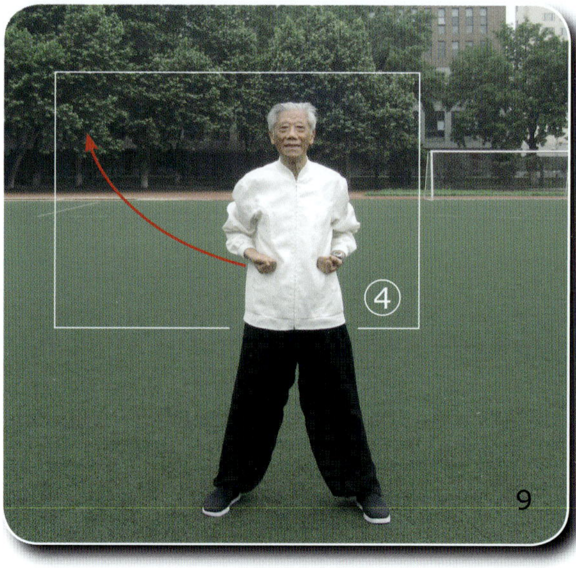

9

3. — 4. Die gleichen Bewegungen wie 1 — 2 in die entgegengesetzte Richtung ausführen. Die Position 2 ist die Ausgangsstellung für die Position 3 (d.h. die Position der Füße wird nicht verändert). Siehe Bilder 6 - 9.

5. — 8. Die gleichen Bewegungen 1 — 4 werden wiederholt.
Die Bewegungen 1 — 8 zweimal oder viermal abwechselnd nach links und rechts ausführen.

Am Ende der Übung die Hände wieder zur Körperseite bringen. Siehe Bild 10.

Anforderungen: Beim Aufrichten der Handflächen und beim Ballen der Faust leichte Kraft benutzen. Mit der gesamten Fußsohle den Kontakt zum Boden halten. Mit weit geöffneten Augen auf die Handfläche blicken und natürlich atmen.

3. — 4. The same movements as in 1 — 2 are carried out in the opposite direction. The last position of sequel 2 is the initial position of sequel 3 (meaning that the position of your feet is not changed). See illustrations 6 - 9.

5. — 8. The same movements 1 — 4 are repeated.
Carry out the movements 1 — 8 two or four times to the left or to the right hand side by turns.

At the end of the exercise guide your hands back to the sides of your body. See illustration 10.

Requirements: When putting your palm upright and when making a fist use slight power only. Keep contact to the ground with the entire soles of your feet. Gaze at your palm with your eyes wide open and breathe naturally.

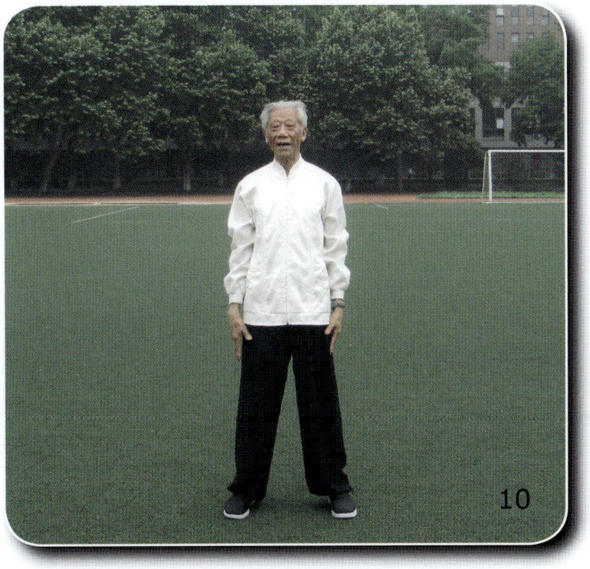

10

## 第八段　七颠诸病消

预备姿势：两脚自然开立，双臂垂于体侧。（图1）

动作：

第一个8拍（呼）：

1—4拍，当双手向前摆起时，双足跟提起；当双手落于体侧时（手心向下），双足跟迅速震地（两脚伸直），一起一震为颠动一次（为一拍），（图2，3）。共做四拍。

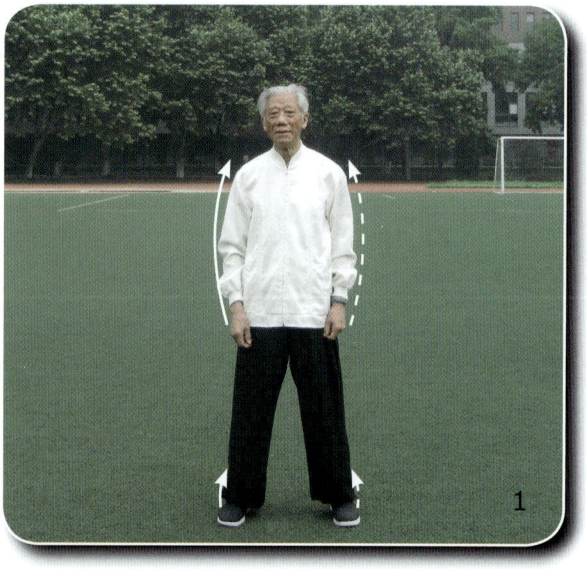

1

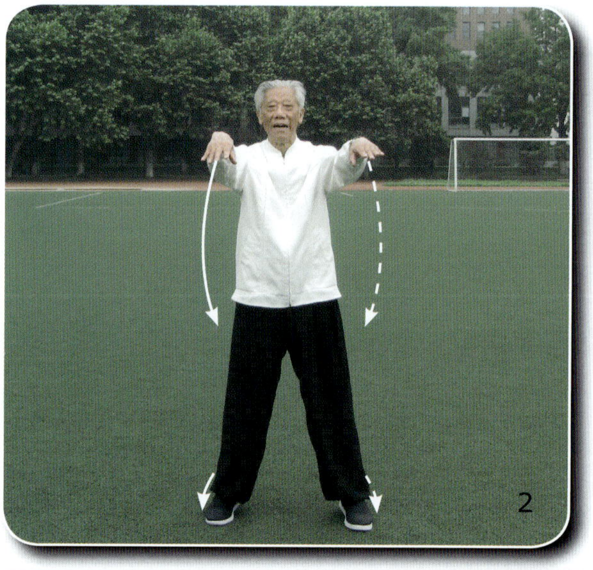

2

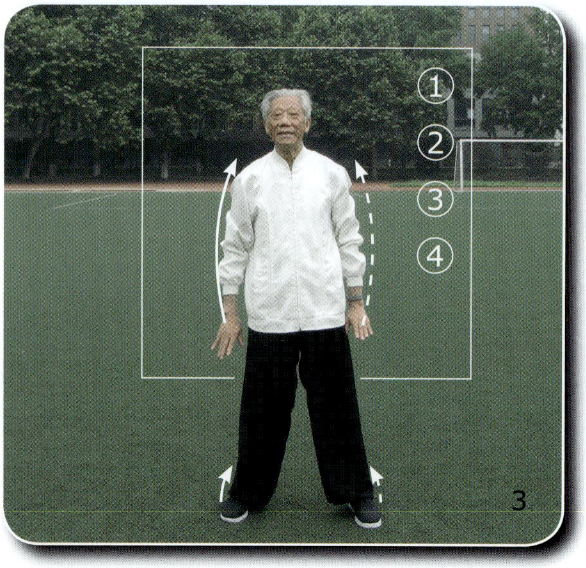


3

## VIII. Sieben Mal rütteln und hundert Krankheiten vertreiben

Ausgangsstellung
Die Füße parallel stellen, schulterbreit auseinander. Die Arme hängen an den Seiten des Körpers. Siehe Bild 1.

Teil 1: 1. — 4. Die Hände schwingen nach vorne, die Fersen dabei vom Boden lösen und anheben. Während die Hände herunterfallen (Handflächen nach unten), die Fersen fallenlassen und die Erde dadurch zum Beben bringen. Die Füße bleiben dabei gestreckt. Siehe Bilder 2 und 3. Insgesamt vier Takte ausführen.

Ein Takt (einmal rütteln) besteht aus einmal anheben und einmal beben.

## VIII. Shaking Seven Times and Expelling a Hundred Illnesses

Initial position
Put your feet parallel, a shoulder breadth apart from each other. Your arms dangle at the sides of your body. See illustration 1.

Part 1: 1. — 4. Your hands swing forewards while you take your heels off the ground and lift them. See illustration 2. While your hands drop (palms downwards), make the ground quake by quickly dropping your heels. Your feet remain stretched in doing so. See illustrations 2 and 3. All in all you carry out four beats.

One beat (shaking once) consists of lifting once and quaking once.

5—8拍，双手改为向左右摆起和落于体侧，双足动作与1—4相同。（图4—6）

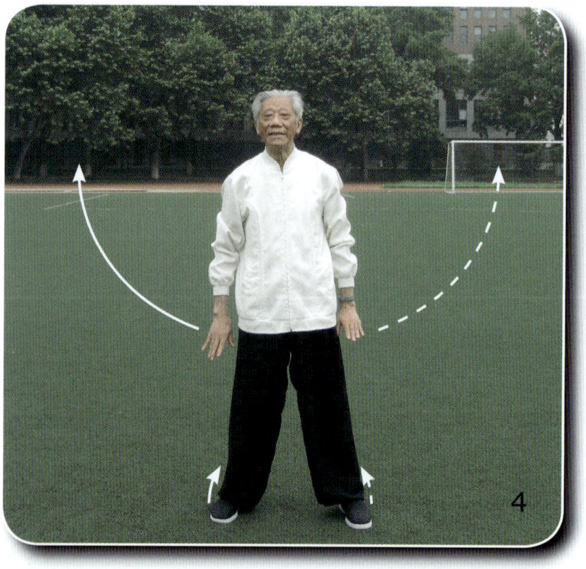


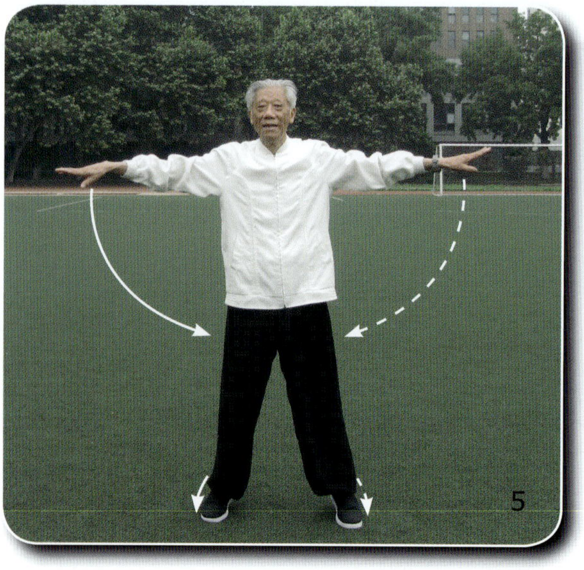


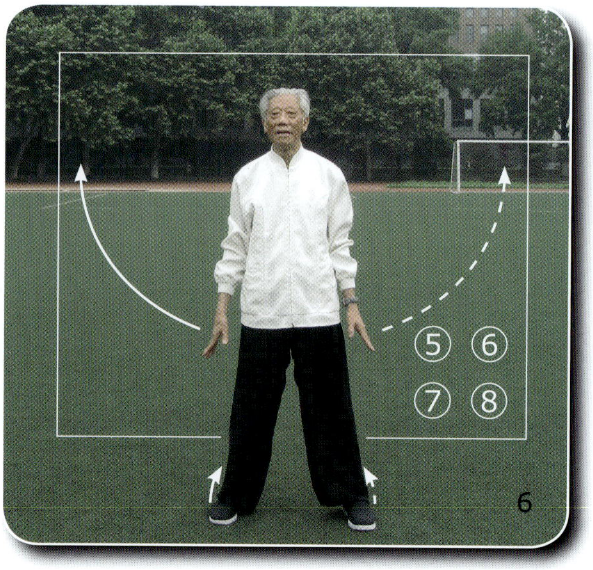

5. — 8. Die Hände schwingen zu den Seiten, die Fersen dabei vom Boden lösen und anheben. Siehe Bilder 4 und 5. Anschließend die Hände und Fersen fallen lassen. Die Beine bleiben dabei gestreckt. Siehe Bild 6. Insgesamt vier Takte ausführen.

Ein Takt (einmal rütteln) besteht aus einmal anheben und einmal beben.

5. — 8. Your hands swing to your sides while you take your heels off the ground and lift them. See illustrations 4 and 5. After this you drop your hands and your heels. In doing so you keep your legs straight. See illustration 6. All in all you carry out four beats.

One beat (shaking once) consists of lifting once and quaking once.

第二个8拍（呼）：

1—4拍，当双手（手心向下）由里向前向外划平圆时，双足跟提起。当双手由外向里划圆时，双足跟迅速震地，一起一震为颠动一次（为一拍），（图1—3）。共做四拍。

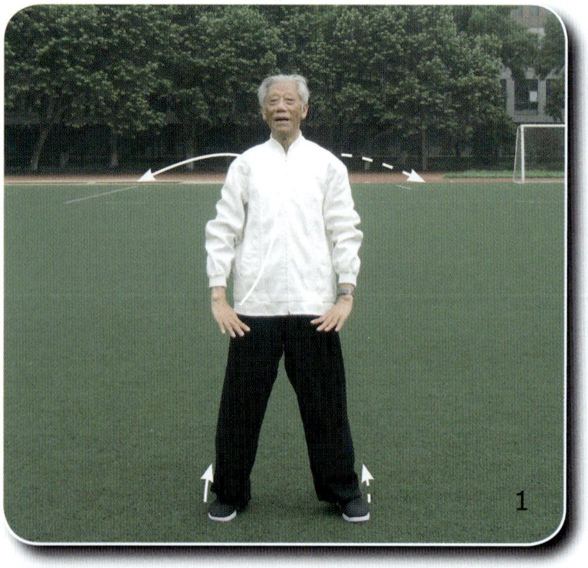


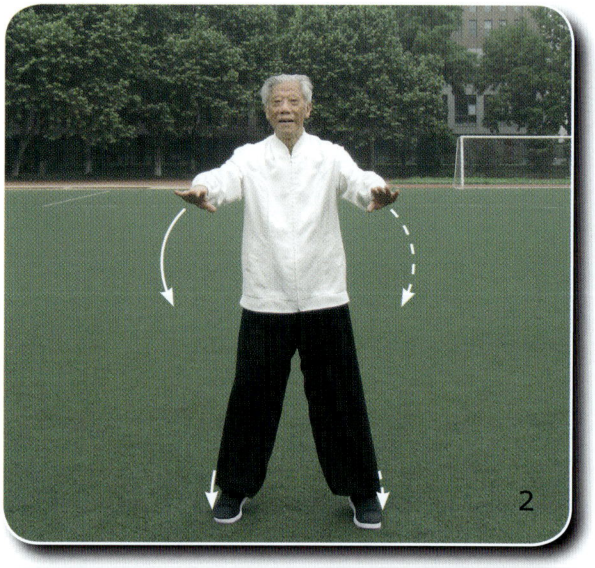


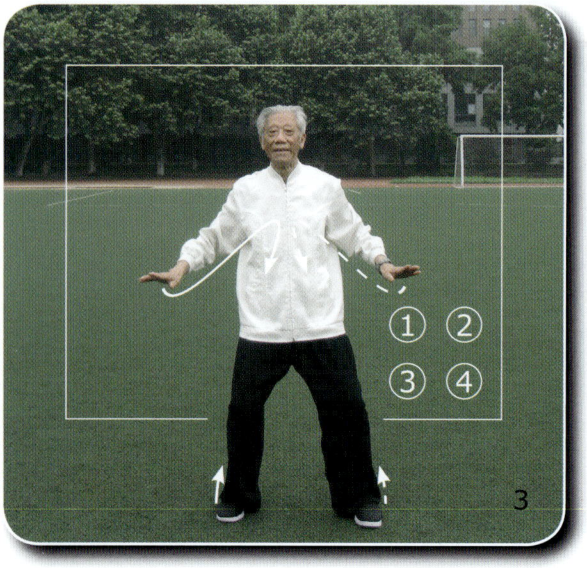

Teil 2:
1. — 4. Die Hände (Handflächen nach unten) in einer kreisförmigen Bewegung nach vorne und außen bringen (eine ähnliche Bewegung wie beim Schwimmen). Die Fersen dabei vom Boden lösen und anheben. Während die Hände wieder von außen nach innen in einer kreisförmigen Bewegung zurückgebracht werden, fallen die Fersen schnell zu Boden und bringen die Erde dadurch zum Beben. (Die Beine bleiben dabei gestreckt). Siehe Bilder 1 - 3. Insgesamt vier Takte ausführen.

Part 2:
1. — 4. Guide your hands (palms downwards) to the front and outwards in a circular movement (a movement similar to swimming). In doing so take your heels off the ground and lift them. While you guide your hands back again in a circular movement from their outward position inwards, your heels drop to the ground quickly and make the ground quake. (In doing so your legs remain straight). Illustrations 1 - 3. All in all you carry out four beats.

5—8拍，双手划圆的方向反，双足动作与1—4相同。（图4—6）

练习次数：共做两个八拍，结束时，双手由外向里合抱重叠于丹田。
（男性左手在里，右手在外，女性方向相反。）

要求：颠动时宜震动全身，注意放松，自然呼吸。

## 收功:

搓手，浴面，梳头，捏耳朵，揉风池，揉两肾。

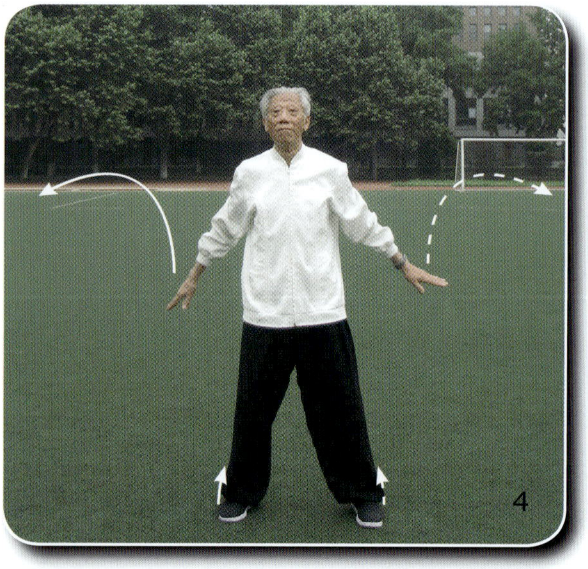
4

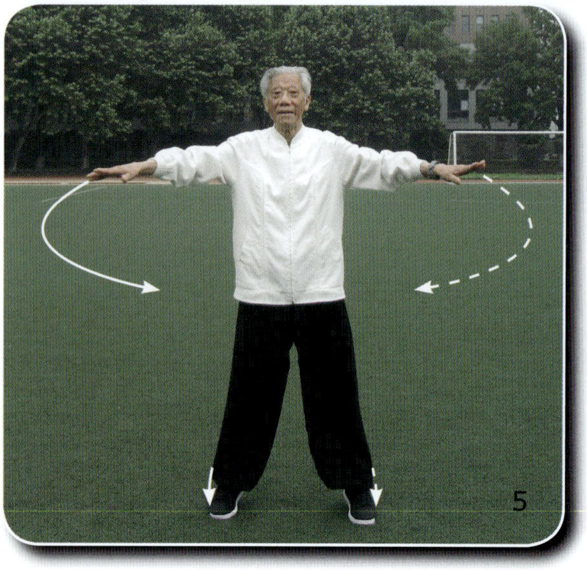
5

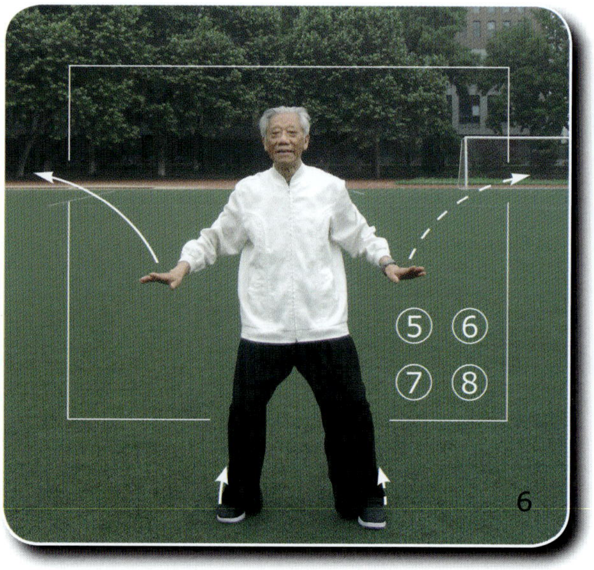

6

5. — 8. Dieselbe Fußbewegung wie 1. — 4., nur die Hände in die entgegengesetzte Richtung kreisen. Siehe Bilder 4 - 6.
Die Übung (Teile 1 und 2) einmal komplett ausführen.

Am Ende der Übung die Hände von außen nach innen auf das untere DanTian (Energiezentrum des Körpers) etwa 3,5 cm unterhalb des Bauchnabels aufeinander legen. (Die Frauen legen zuerst die rechte Hand, dann die linke Hand auf. Die Männer machen es umgekehrt).

Anforderungen: Beim Rütteln mit dem ganzen Körper beben. Dabei darauf achten, mit dem ganzen Körper zu entspannen. Natürlich atmen.

## Abschlußübung

Die Hände aneinanderlegen und die Handflächen reiben. Mit den Handflächen das Gesicht massieren, vom Kinn aus über Nase und Stirn zu den Wangen und zurück zum Kinn. Mit sanftem Druck mit den Fingerspitzen die Haare kämmen, vom Haaransatz bis zum Nacken. Mit Daumen und Zeigefinger die Ohren massieren. Mit den Fingerspitzen den Punkt FengChi links und rechts am Hinterkopf massieren. Zum Abschluß mit den Händen zu den Nieren gehen und sie massieren.

5. — 8. The same movement of your feet as in 1. — 4., but you make your hands circle in the opposite direction. See illustrations 4 - 6.
Carry out the exercise (parts 1 and 2) one time completely.

At the end of the exercise put your hands on each other from their outward position inwards onto the nether Dan Tian (energy centre of the body), approximately 3,5 cm underneath your navel. (Women put their right hand first, then their left hand. Men carry this out in the opposite way).

Requirements: When shaking quake with your entire body. In doing so mind that you relax your entire body. Breathe naturally.

## Final Exercise

Put your palms next to each other and rub them. Massage your face with your palms, starting from your chin, passing your nose and forehead, advancing towards your cheeks and back to your chin. Comb your hair with soft pressure with your fingertips from your forehead to the back of your neck. Massage your ears with your thumbs and indexfingers. Massage FengChi Point with your fingertips at the right and left hand sides of the back of your neck. Finally guide your hands to your kidneys and massage them.

## 练习动作全图

## Übersicht der Übungen



## Survey of the Exercises

## 第一段　托天理三焦

## I. Mit den Händen den Himmel stützen und den Dreifachen-Erwärmer-Meridian ausrichten

## I. Supporting Heaven with Your Hands, Straighten the Triple–Warmer-Meridian

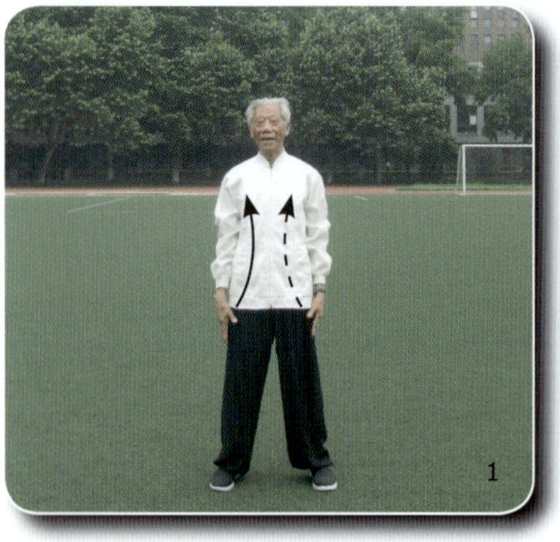


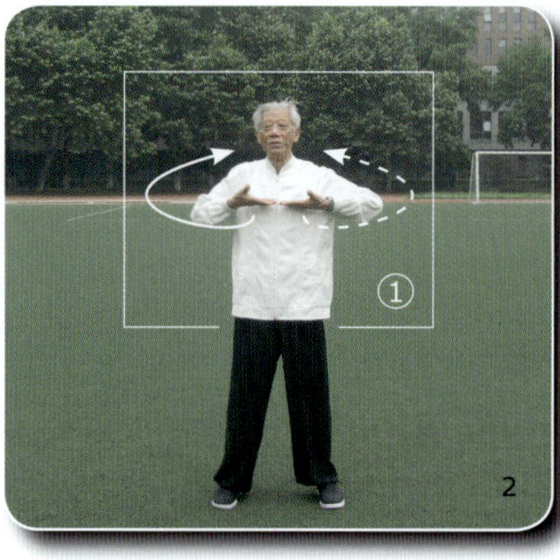


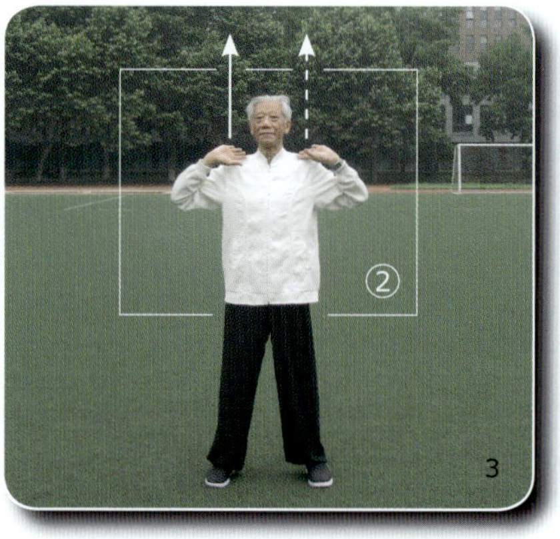


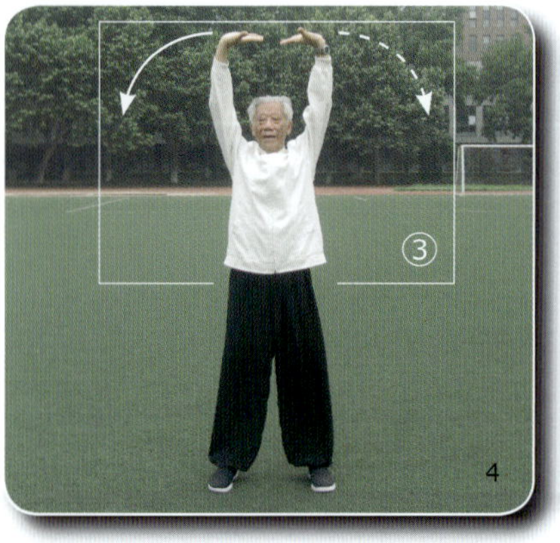


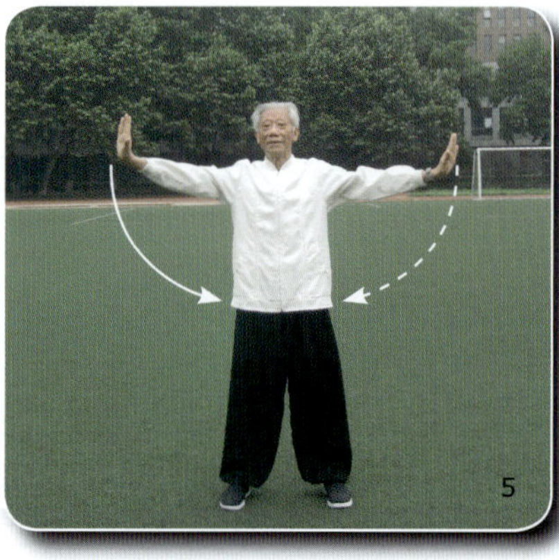


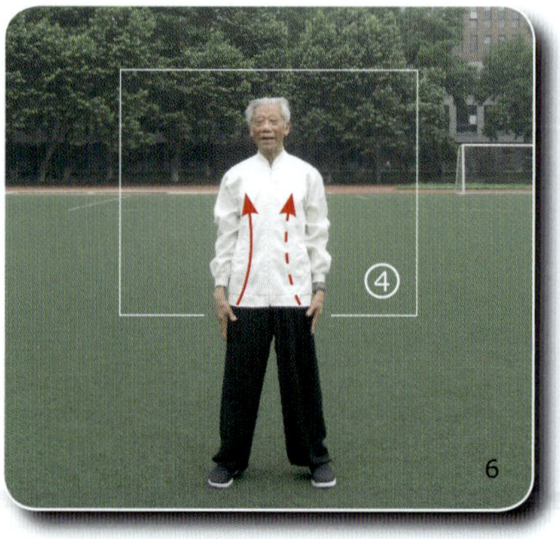

## 第二段　拉弓似射雕
## II. Den Bogen spannen und auf den Geier zielen
## II. Drawing the Bow and Aiming at the Vulture

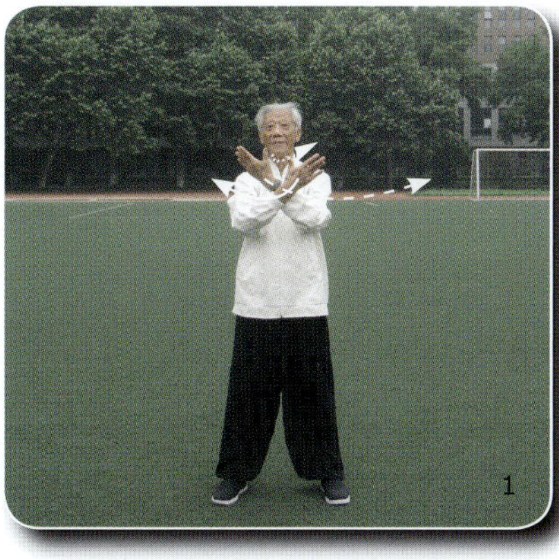


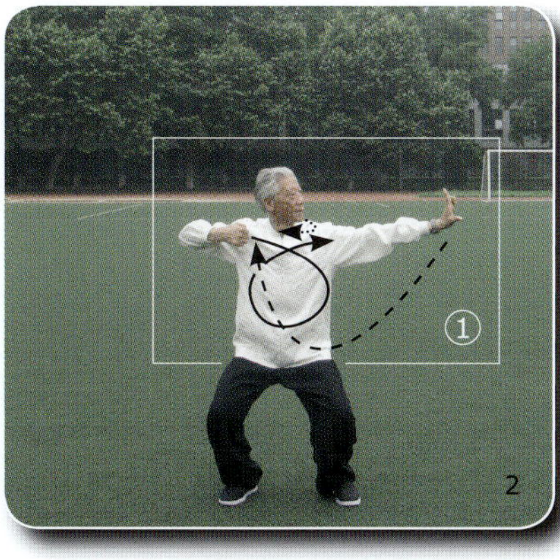


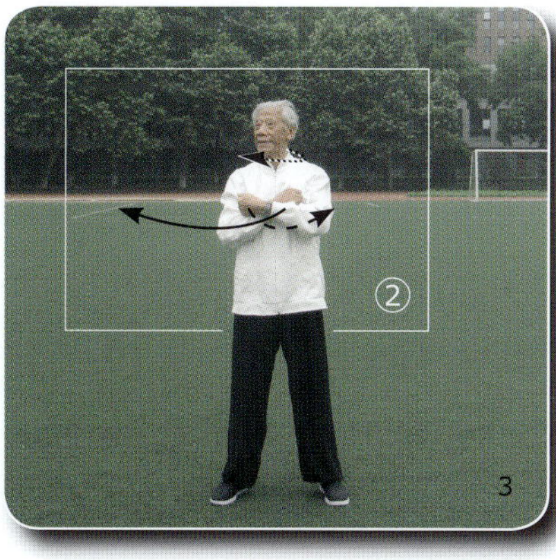


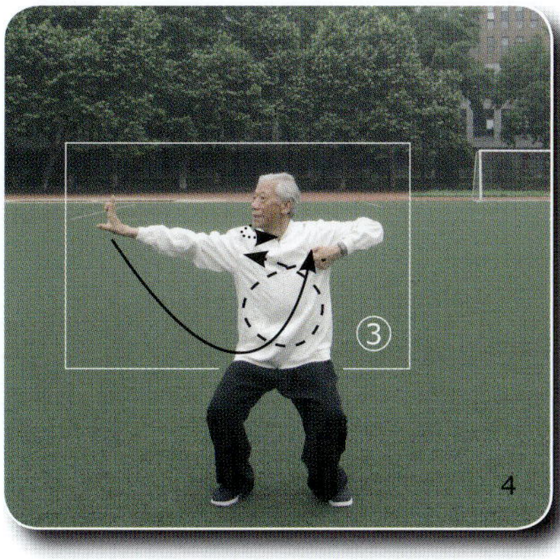


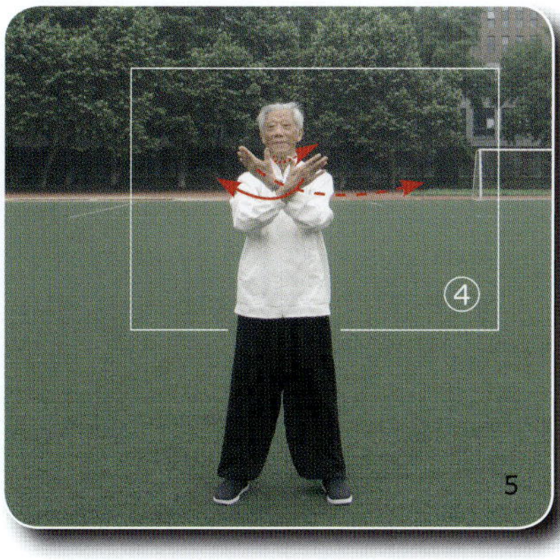

## 第三段　单举健脾胃

III. Die Arme einzeln hochheben, um Magen und Milz zu regulieren

III. Lift Your Arms One by One to Regulate Your Stomach and Your Spleen

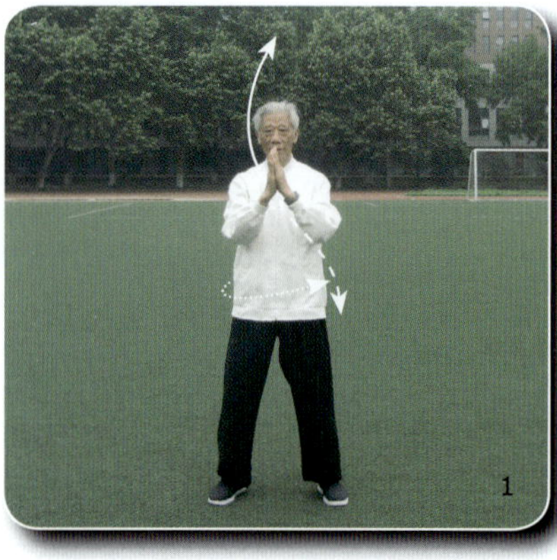


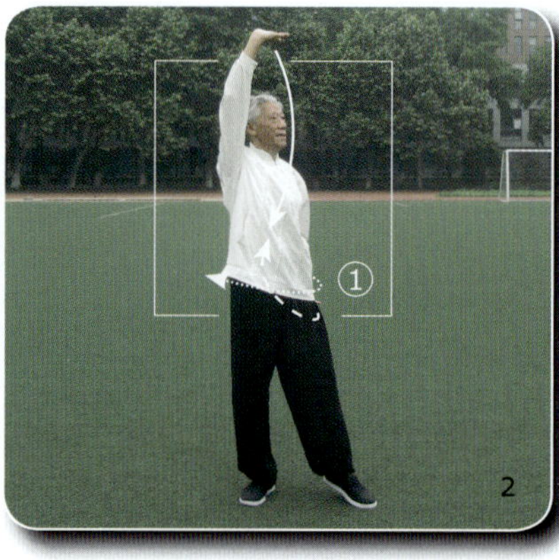


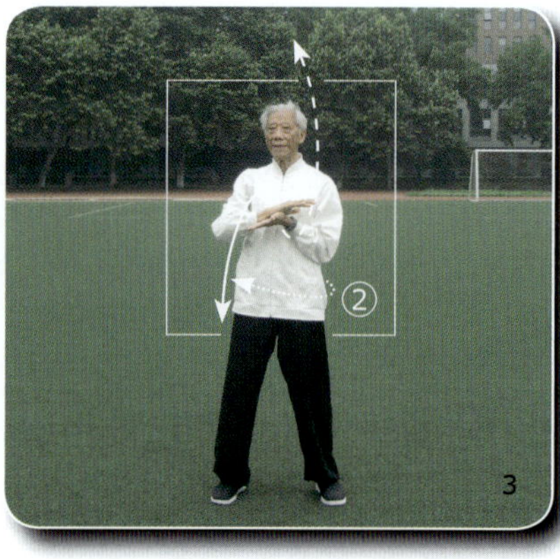


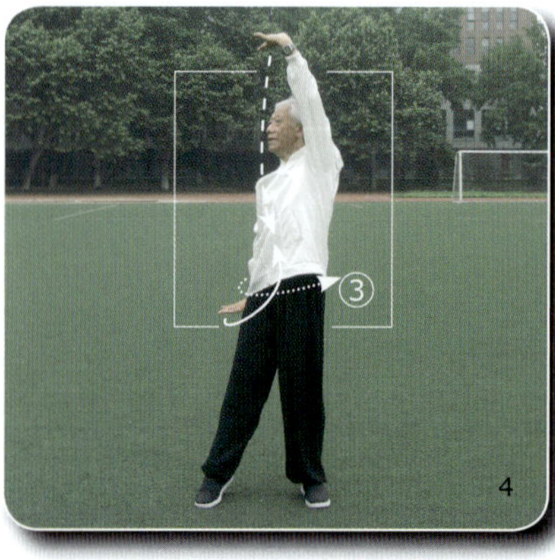


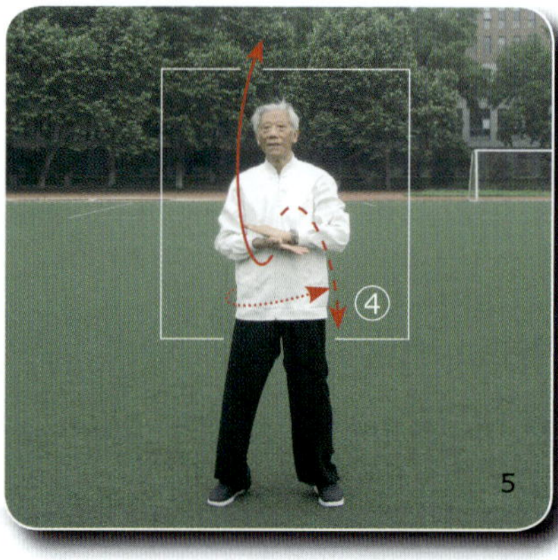

## 第四段　劳伤向后瞧

## IV. Die von den Fünf Anstrengungen und Sieben Betrübnissen verursachten Krankheiten vertreiben

## IV. Expel the Illnesses Caused by the Five Strains and the Seven Afflictions

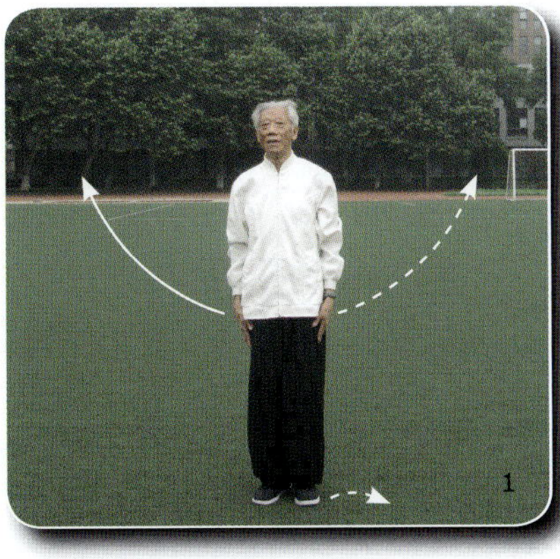


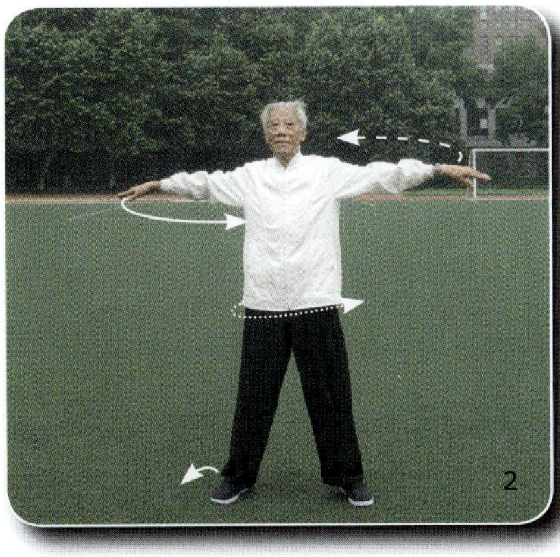


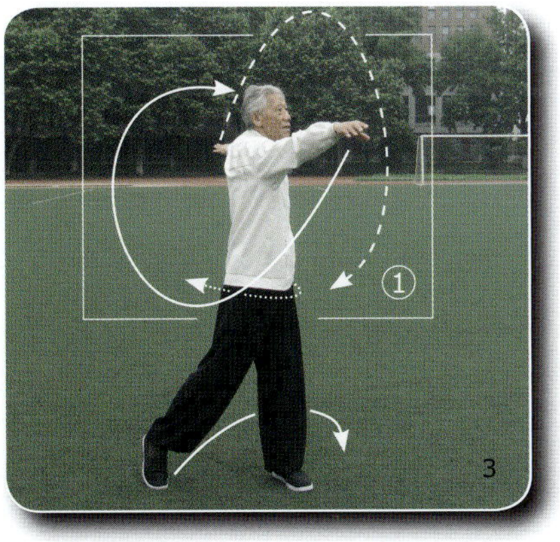


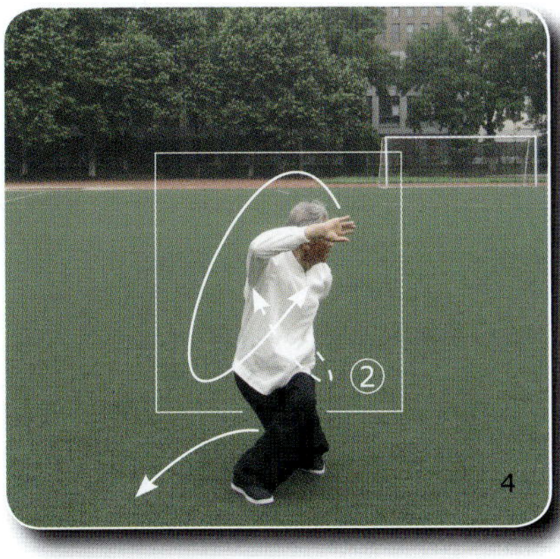


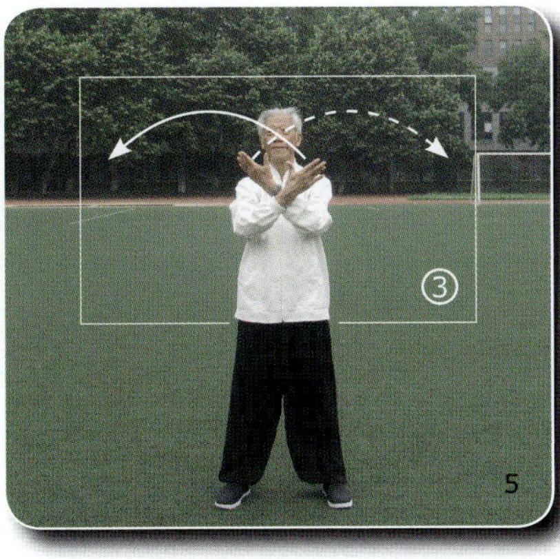


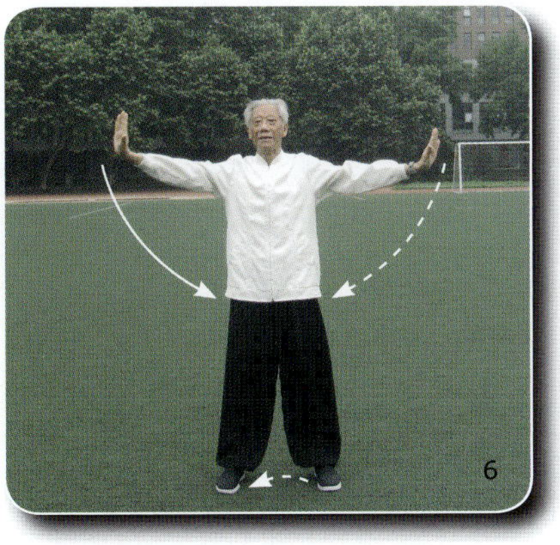


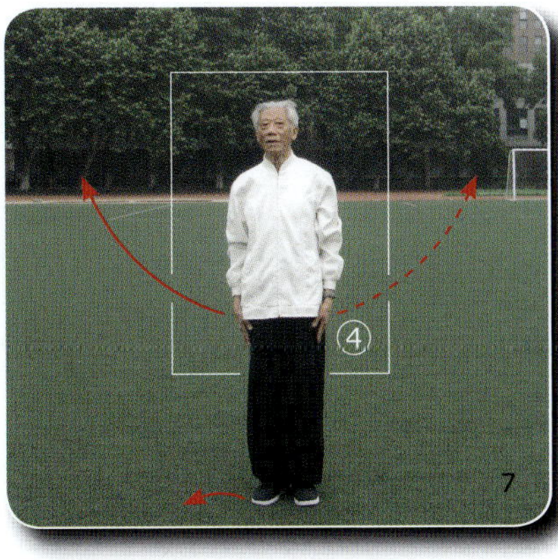

## 第五段　摇摆去心火

## V. Mit Wiegen und Wedeln die innere Hitze aus dem Herzen vertreiben

## V. Expel the Inner Heat from Your Heart by Rocking and Wagging

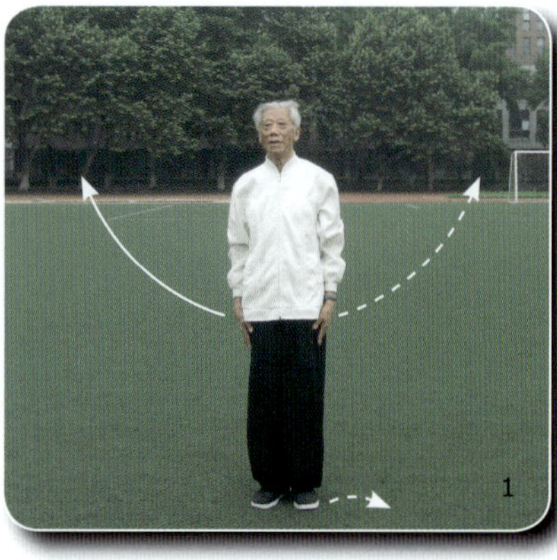


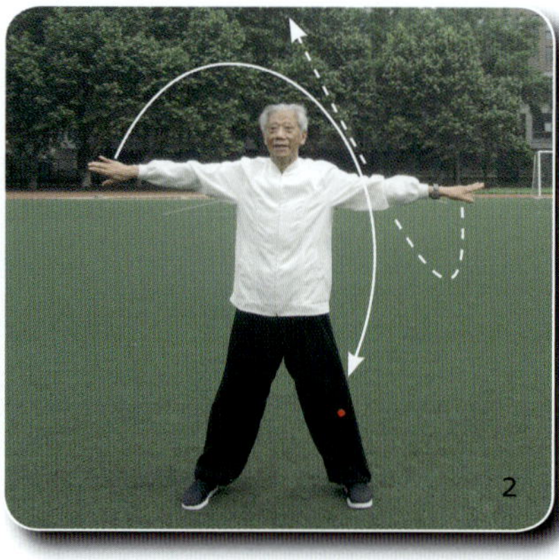


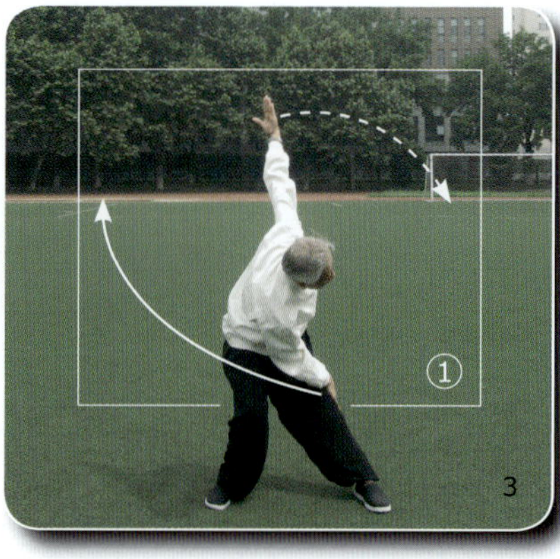


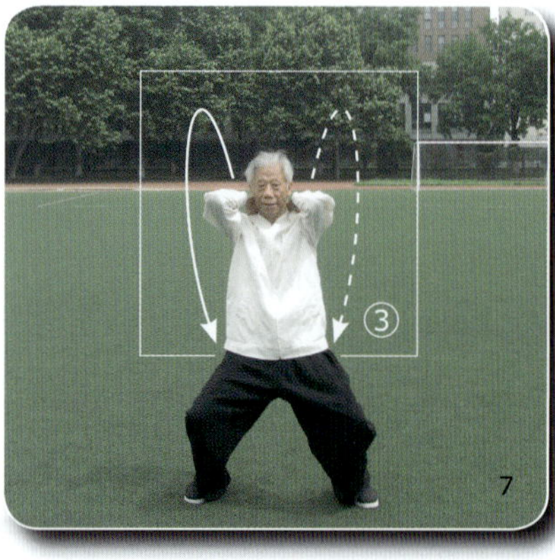


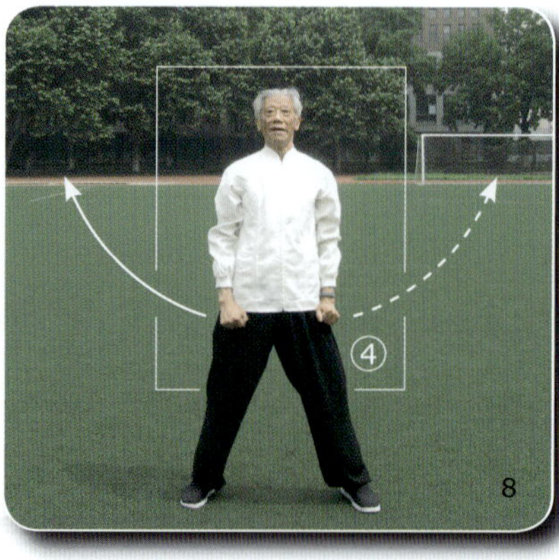


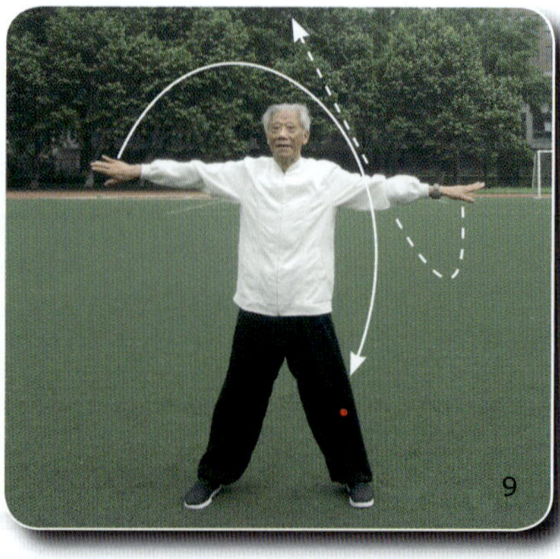


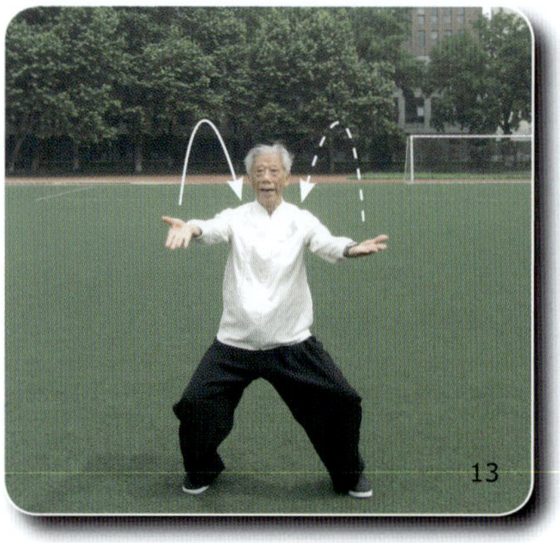


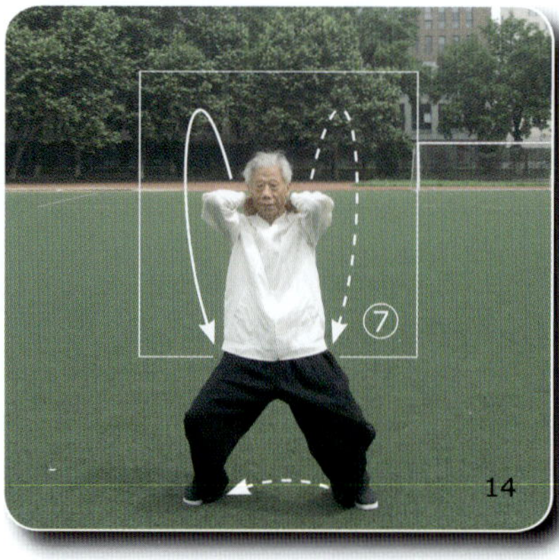


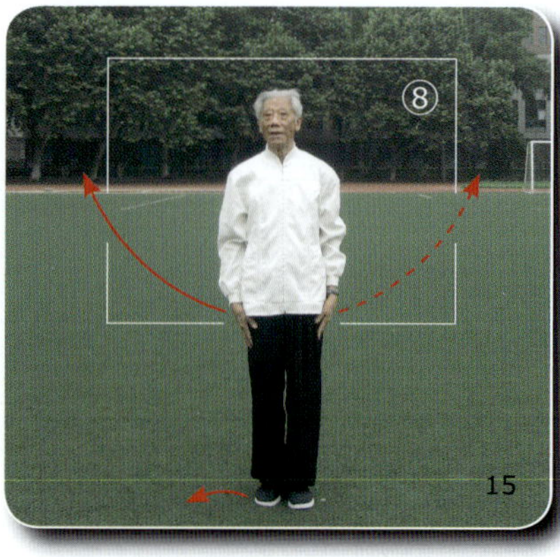

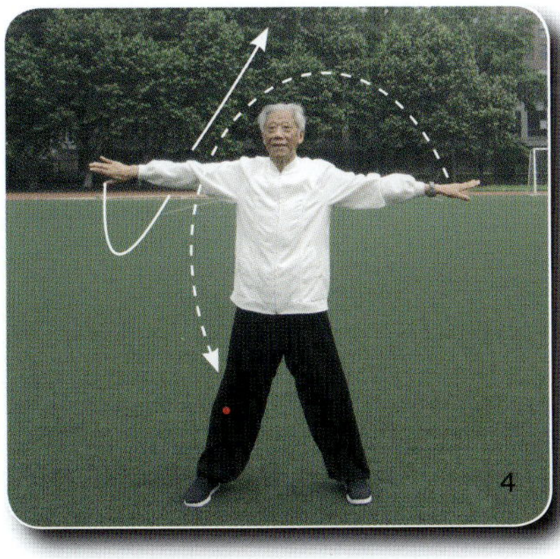
4

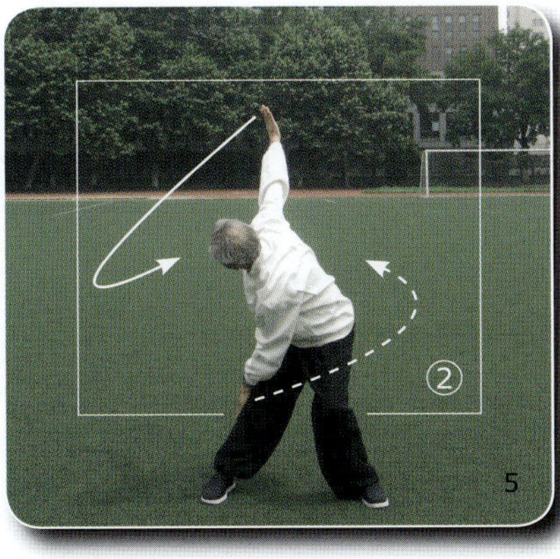
②
5

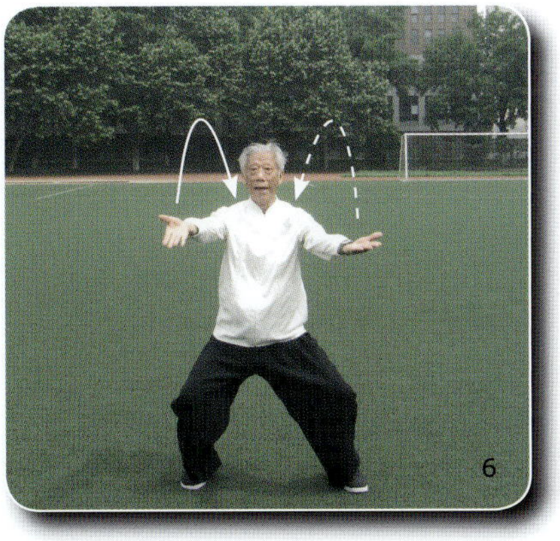
6

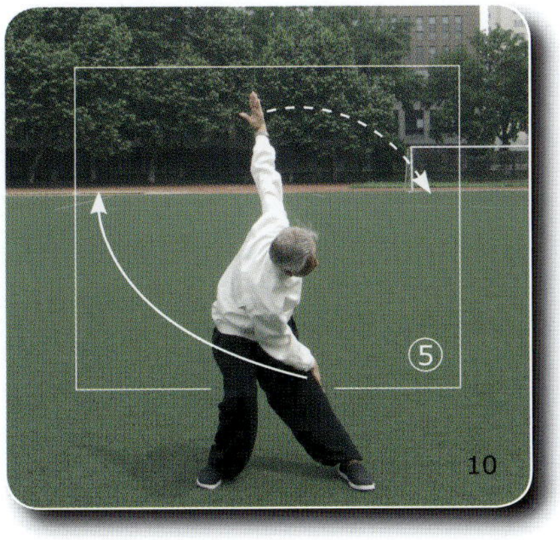
⑤
10

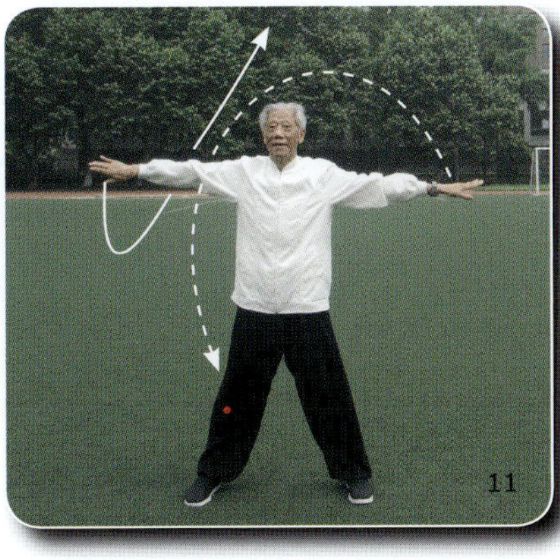
11

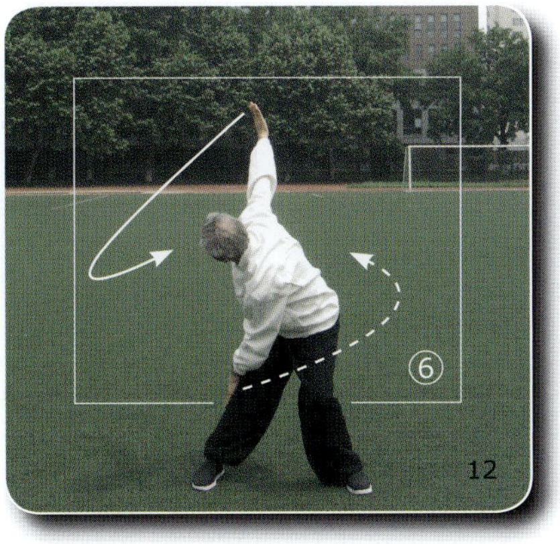
⑥
12

## 第六段　躬身固肾腰
## VI. Tief beugen, um die Nieren und den Hüftbereich zu stärken
## VI. Bend Deep Down to Strengthen Your Kidneys and the Region of Your Hips

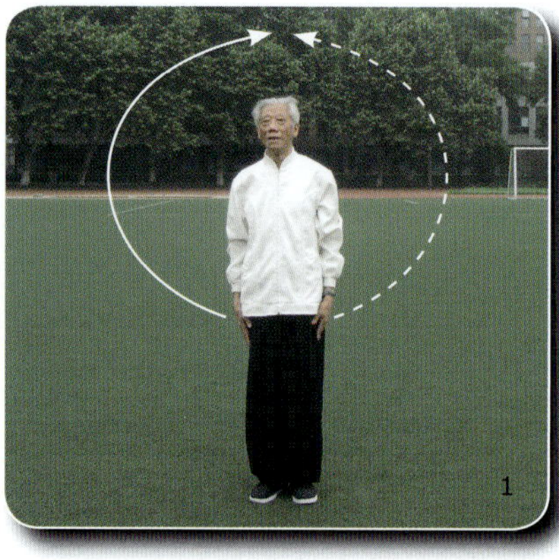


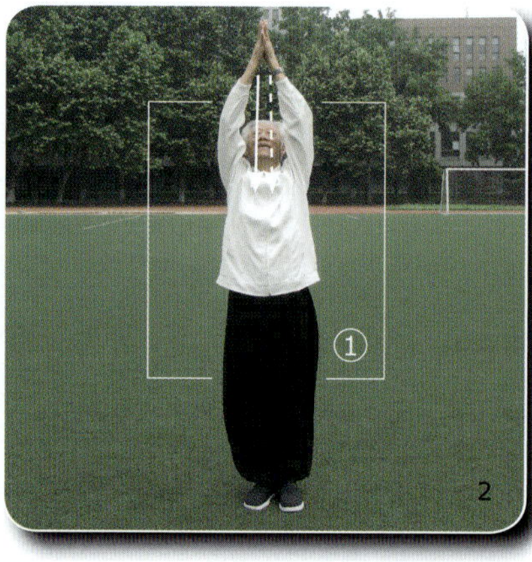


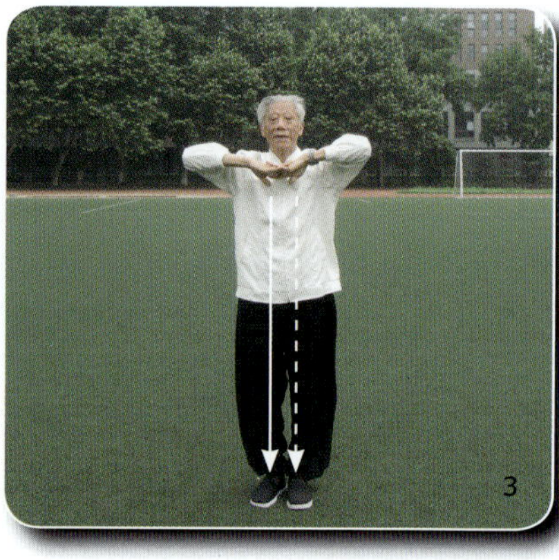


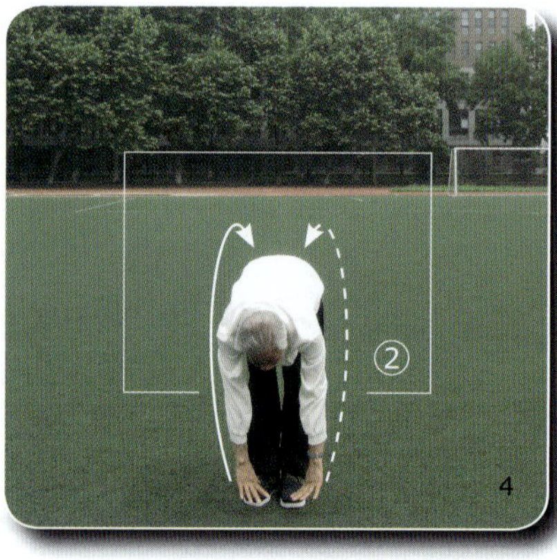


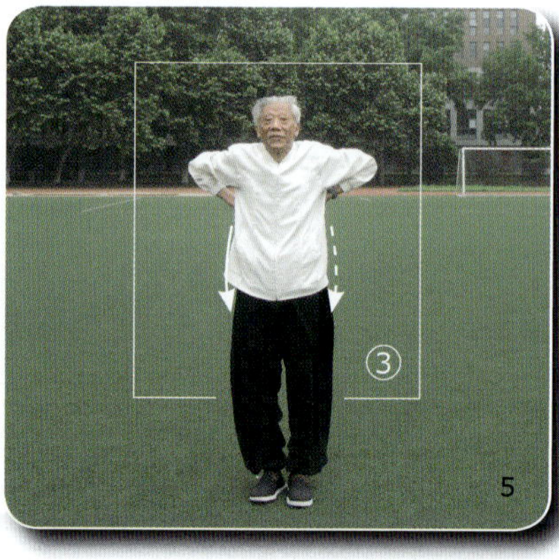


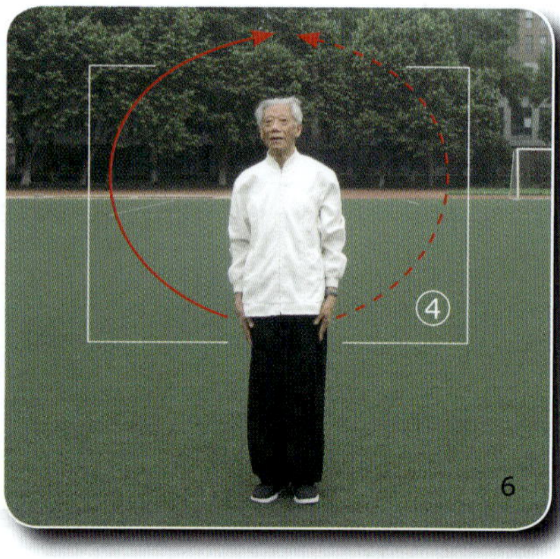

## 第七段　瞪目增气力

## VII. Die Augen weit öffnen – Qi vermehren

## VII. Open Your Eyes Wide – Enhancing Qi

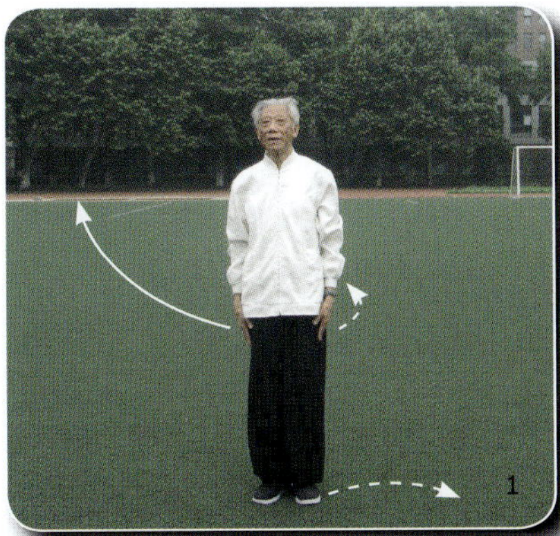


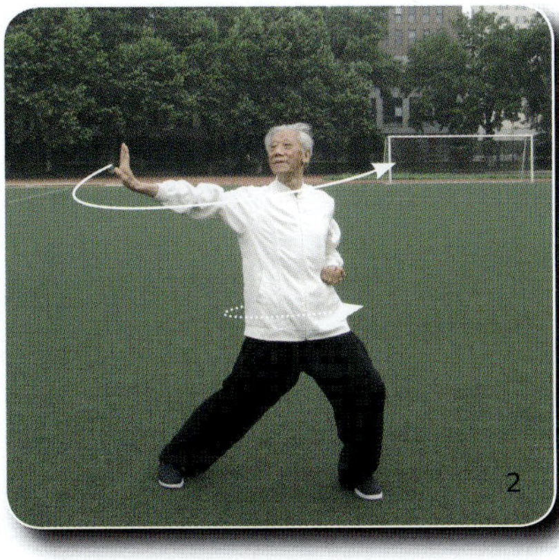


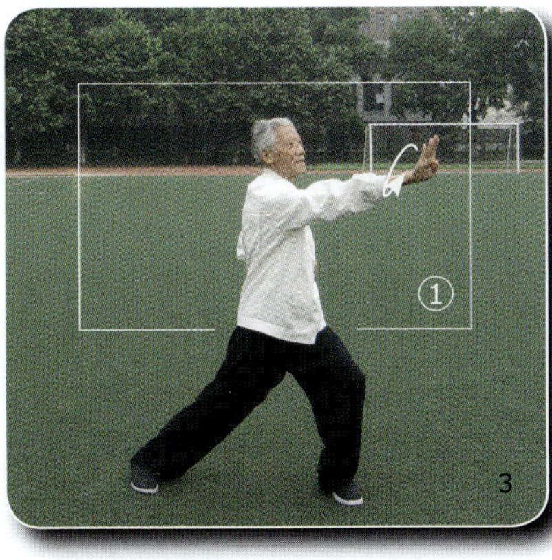


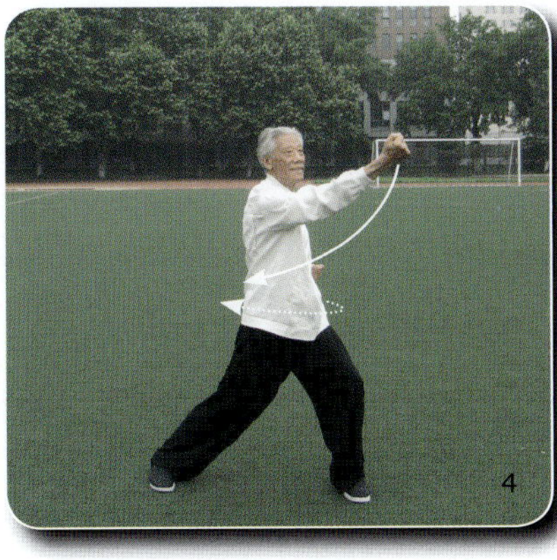


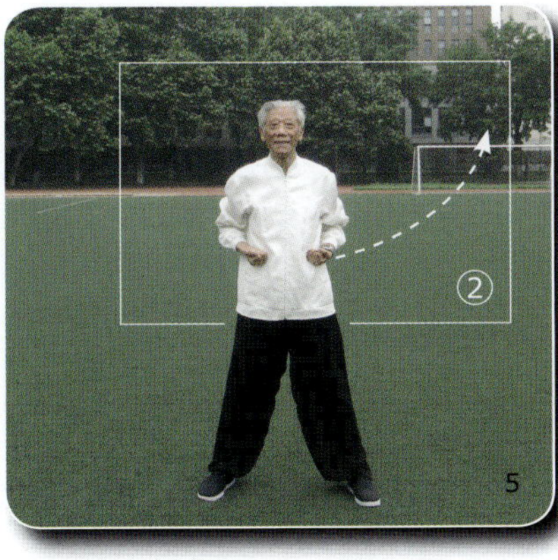


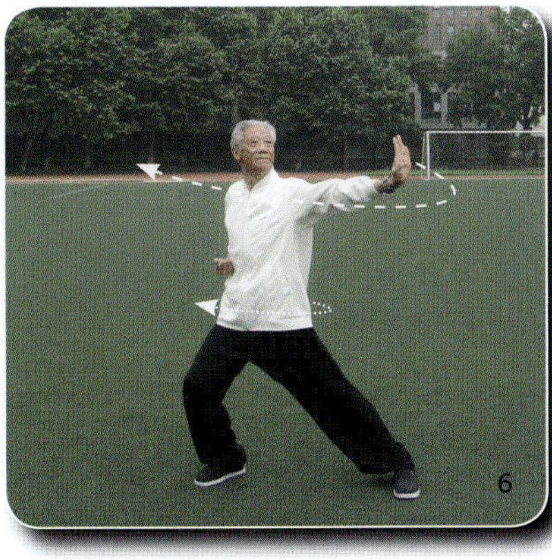


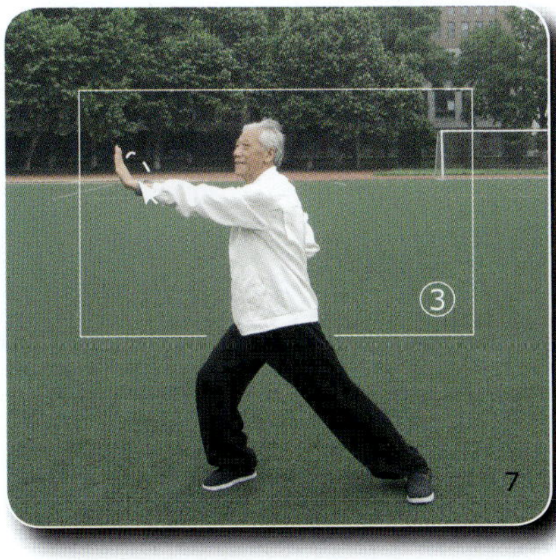


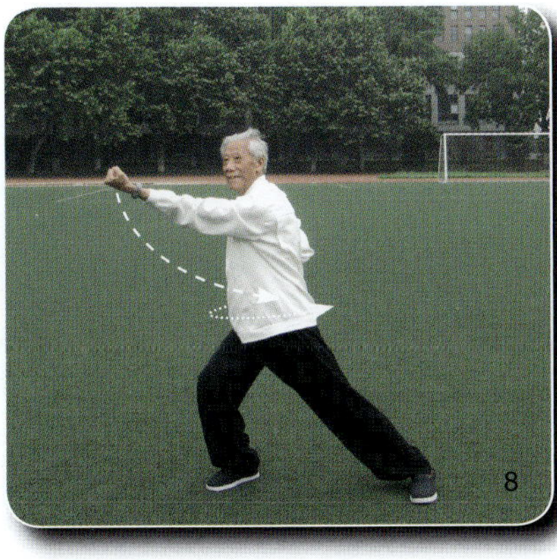


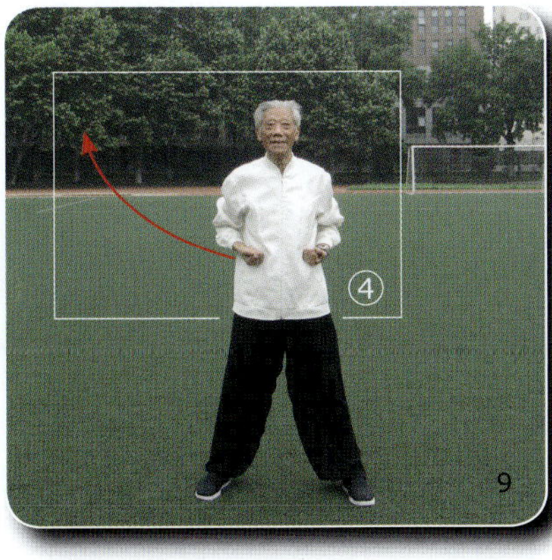

## 第八段　七颠诸病消

### 第一个8拍

### VIII. Sieben Mal rütteln und hundert Krankheiten vertreiben　Teil 1

### VIII. Shaking Seven Times and Expelling a Hundred Illnesses　Part 1

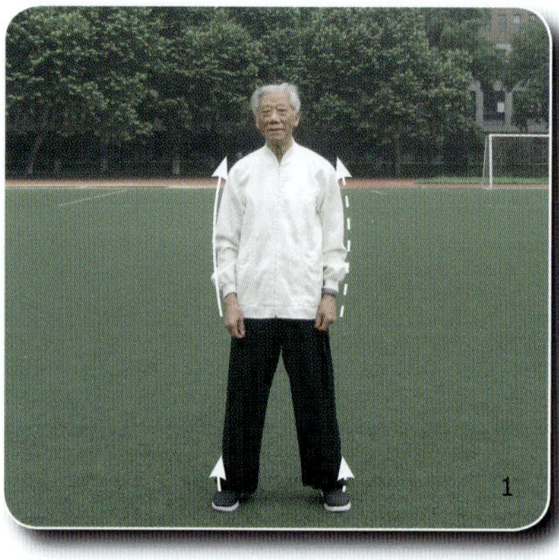


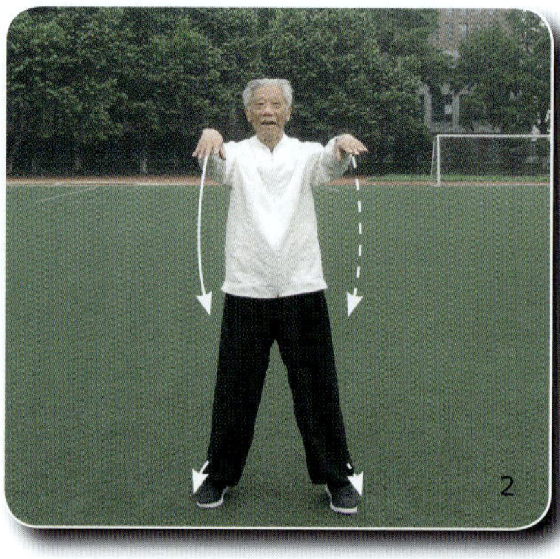


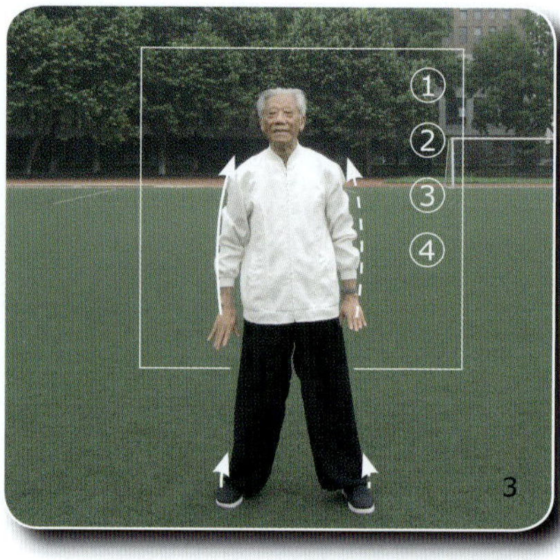


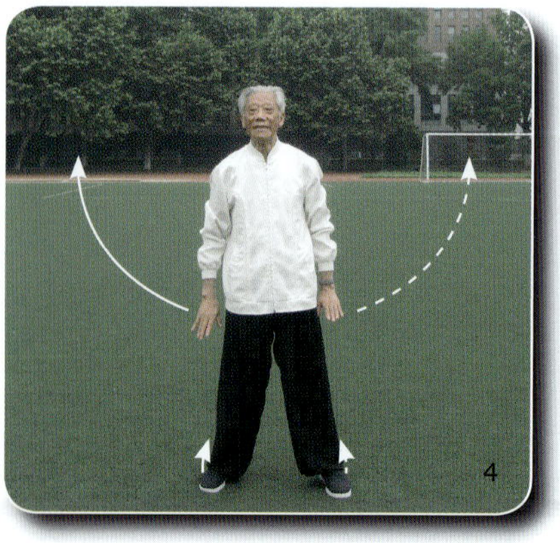


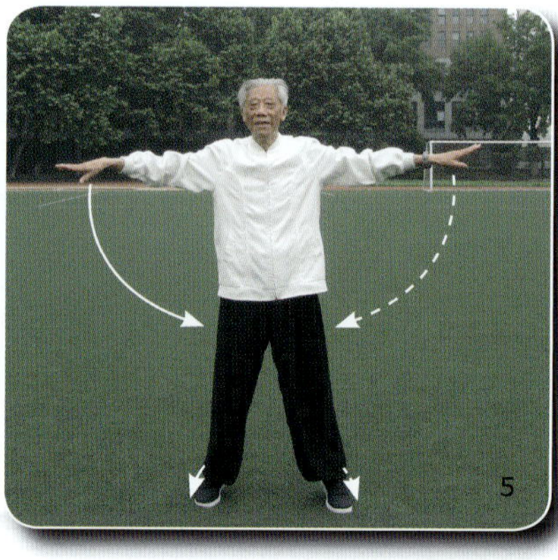


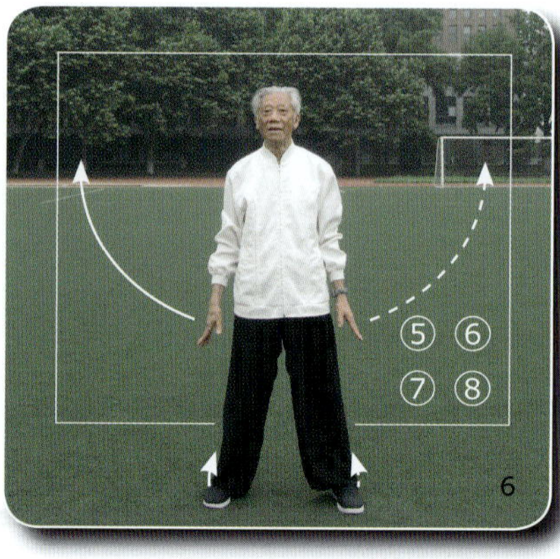

## 第八段　七颠诸病消

### 第二个8拍

### VIII. Sieben Mal rütteln und hundert Krankheiten vertreiben　Teil 2

### VIII. Shaking Seven Times and Expelling a Hundred Illnesses　Part 2

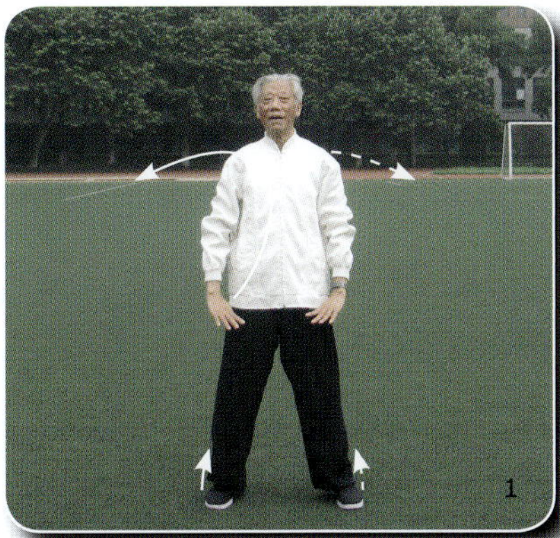


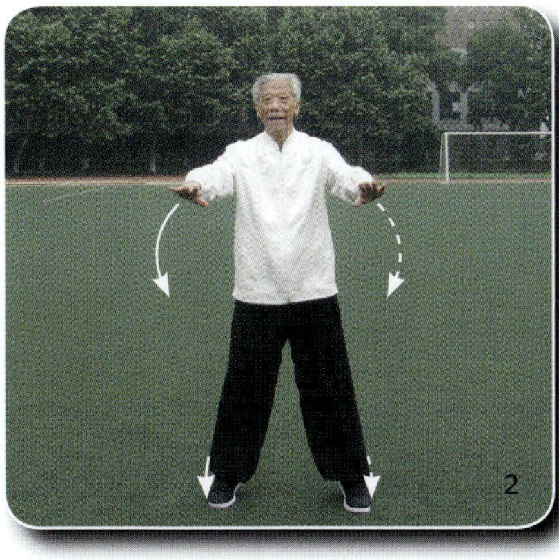


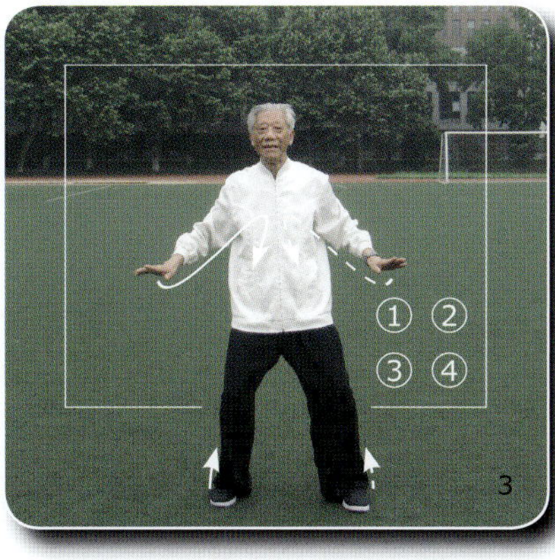


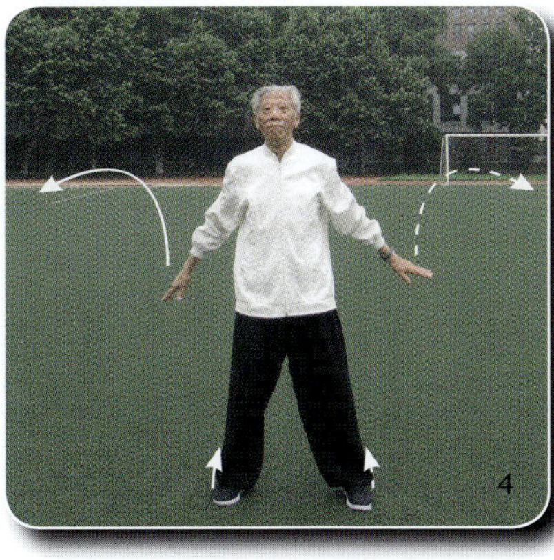


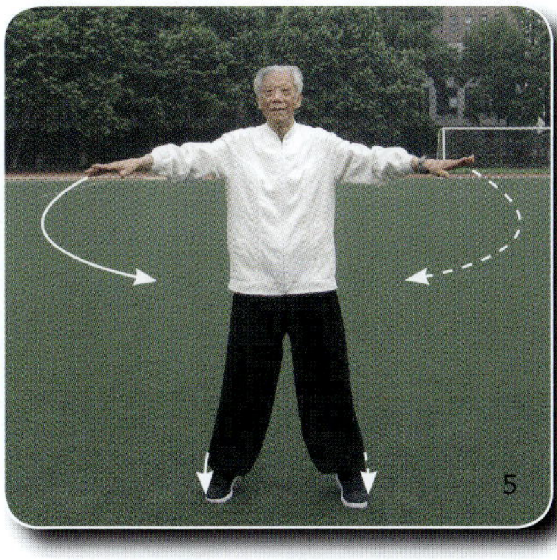


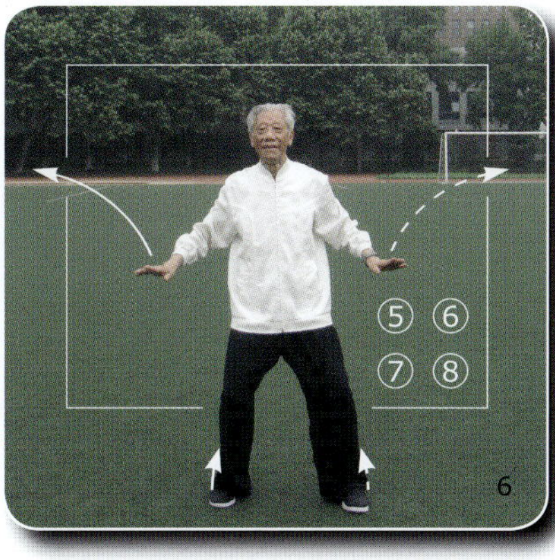

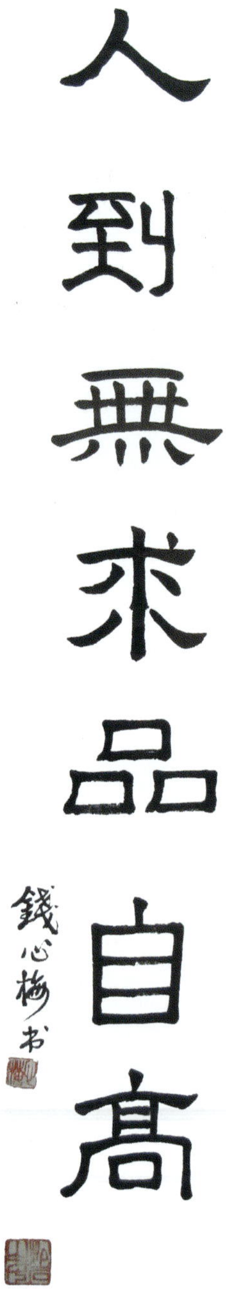


Wenn man keine Forderungen hat,
erreicht der Charakter ein hohes Niveau...

If you do not have any expectations,
your character may reach a high level...

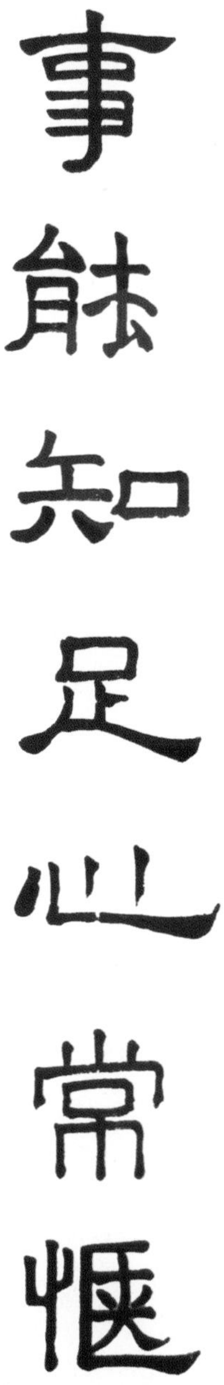


Bleibe bescheiden, besitze die Fähigkeit der Zufriedenheit,
dann werden die Herzenswünsche nicht zu groß...

Stay modest, possess the ability of contentment,
then your heartfelt wishes will not become too big...

Calligraphy by Qian XinMei 钱心梅. Yan Gronau is the daughter of Qian XinMei. She lives in Germany and is considered an expert in traditional Chinese painting and calligraphy. www.yan-gronau.de

# 拉筋正骨功　丁宏余

（简称：筋骨功）

拉筋正骨功，它是一种全身性的运动，是为中老年朋友‘抗衰延寿、延长生活自理能力’而编制的。筋与骨是一对同胞兄弟，两者互补、互依、同存……。人体的一切活动（动作），全靠它们（加上肌肉）的功能协调发挥来完成的。筋，要求能拉长、能收紧，富有弹性。骨，要求坚固、强硬，能承受较大压力。关节活动，显得灵活自如，柔韧性好……。以上种种要求，只有健康的年轻人才能具备。可是人们随着年龄的增加，筋逐渐趋向萎缩，骨逐渐趋向松脆，关节活动受阻，都是老化的表现。

健康问题，务虚（理论）当然需要，可务实更为重要。多数老年人，出现弓腰驼背、两腿没劲、走路不稳、双手无力、伸直困难，关节活动受阻等等。祖国医学认为：骨正筋柔，气血自流，经络畅通，身无疼痛；“筋长一寸，延寿十年”，是内经中的名言。因此，平时注重拉筋、强骨活动，发展身体柔韧性，就显得尤为重要了。

练功要求：本着“安全第一，缓慢用力，循序渐进，坚持有效”的原则来练习。

2012年5月15日

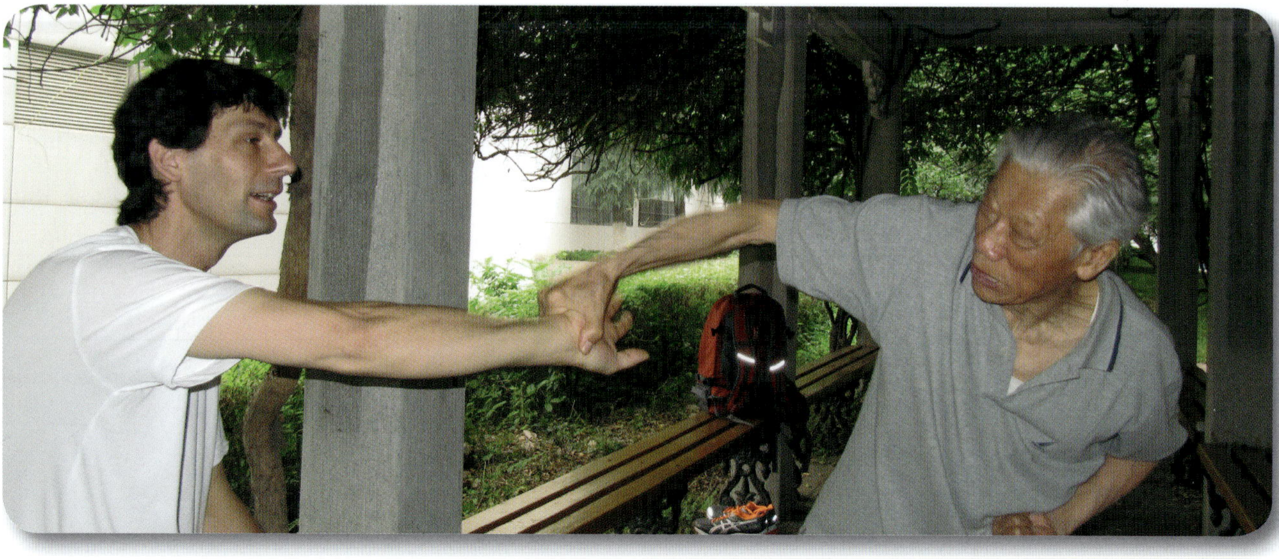

Alexander Callegari－丁宏余教授　2013年

## 注意事项

1、拉筋前做好热身运动，使肌肉、韧带发热后，或微出汗即可进行。

2、动作的力度、幅度、速度、量度以适合自己为最佳。（为保证安全，在练习中不要借用他力或他人帮助，到不到位（指刺激）？过不过头（指疼痛）？只有自己最清楚）

3、不怕起点低，只怕有心人，能坚持就有进步。来日放长，不急于求成。（最好每天练一次，每次20-30分钟左右，有困难者，每周不要少于三次）

4、动作中有绷紧，有放松，松紧结合，有时绷紧的时间要长一些，放松的时间短一些，但要把‘松’贯穿于始终（某一种练习后，也要放松）。这样练的肌肉质量较高，韧带更富有弹性。

5、呼吸要求：第一和第九节动作可以采用自然呼吸（先吸后呼）。第二到第六节和第八节采用一拍吸一拍呼。第七节在放慢速度练习时每拍一吸一呼。

6、本功法可根据需要，选择单项练或全套练。（也可用于集体表演）

7、衣着要宽松柔软。

8、结束后要注意保暖，防止关节受风寒袭击，可适度饮水。

9、发烧、发着关节炎者禁练，腰、腿疼痛，肝、肾不好者慎练，或听取医生的意见。

# Sehnen- und Knochen-QiGong (JinGu Gong)

## Einleitung

Die Sehnen ziehen und dehnen, die Knochen stabilisieren

Das „Sehnen- und Knochen-QiGong" ist eine Sportart mit systematischer Ganzkörperbewegung. Es ist eigens für Erwachsene und Senioren konzipiert. Ziel ist es, den Alterungsprozeß zu verlangsamen, die Lebensdauer zu verlängern und die Selbständigkeit im Alltagsleben zu verbessern. Sehnen und Knochen sind wie Zwillingsbrüder: Die beiden ergänzen sich gegenseitig, sind voneinander abhängig und existieren gemeinsam. Dank der funktionellen Koordination von Sehnen, Knochen und Muskeln können alle Aktivitäten des menschlichen Körpers (Bewegungen) ausgeführt werden.

Die Sehnen sollen gedehnt, straffgezogen und elastisch sein. Die Knochen sollen stabil, stark und zäh sein und müssen in der Lage sein, Druck zu widerstehen. Die Bewegungen in den Gelenken sollen flexibel und gut ausführbar, die Gelenke biegsam und geschmeidig sein. Die oben genannten Anforderungen können junge Menschen leicht erreichen. Aber mit der natürlichen Alterung schrumpfen die Sehnen langsam, die Knochen werden zerbrechlich und porös. Die Beweglichkeit der Gelenke wird zunehmend gehemmt, blockiert oder verhindert. Viele ältere Menschen haben einen krummen Rücken, ihre Beine und Hände haben keine Kraft mehr, beim Gehen sind sie unsicher und wackelig und haben beim Geradestrecken des Körpers und der Gliedmaßen Schwierigkeiten. Um diese gesundheitlichen Probleme zu lösen, muss man nicht nur die Ursachen für die Erkrankungen wissen, man muss auch selbst aktiv körperlich die Blockaden lösen. Nach der Traditionellen Chinesischen Medizin zirkulieren das Qi (Energie) und das Blut fließend, wenn die Knochen stark und die Sehnen geschmeidig sind. Wenn die Energie- und Blutkanäle frei sind, hat der Körper keine Schmerzen. Ein bekanntes Zitat aus dem „Kanon der inneren Medizin" (NeiJing)[1] sagt: Die Sehnen um ein Cun[2] zu verlängern bedeutet, zehn Lebensjahre zu gewinnen. Daher ist es sehr wichtig, sich öfters zu dehnen, die Knochen zu stärken und die Biegsamkeit und Geschmeidigkeit des Körpers zu trainieren.

Beim Trainieren des „Sehnen- und Knochen-QiGongs" muss man sich Schritt für Schritt mit der Übung vertraut machen. Die Übungen zeigen sich besonders wirksam, wenn man auf Dauer kontinuierlich dabei bleibt.

Professor Ding HongYu   NanJing, 15. Mai 2012

[1] Das NeiJing ist eine Sammlung von 81 Abhandlungen, die in zwei Teilen zusammengefasst sind. Als medizinisches Fachwerk ist es bis heute grundlegend und richtungweisend für die Ausbildung innerhalb der Traditionellen Chinesischen Medizin.

[2] Das Cun ist eine traditionelle chinesische Maßeinheit. Ein Cun hat 3,33 cm.

## Wichtige Punkte für die Übung

1. Vor der Übung die Muskeln und Bänder durch ausreichende leichte Vorbereitungsübungen mobilisieren. Anschließend den Körper durch schnellere und intensivere Bewegungen aufwärmen, so dass man leicht schwitzt.

2. Die Intensität, die Schwingungsweite und die Geschwindigkeit der Übung muss jeder individuell bestimmen und regulieren. Ebenso die Häufigkeit der Wiederholungen. Jeder muss sich seiner persönlichen körperlichen Grenzen bewußt sein.

3. Mit der Übung des „Sehnen- und Knochen-QiGong" kann man jederzeit beginnen. Um einen Fortschritt zu erzielen, sollte die Übung drei Mal pro Woche, 20 bis 30 Minuten, geübt werden. Man kann die Übung auch jeden Tag ausführen und sie so in den alltäglichen Tagesablauf integrieren.

4. Die An- und Entspannung in der Übung soll gut miteinander kombiniert werden. Manchmal soll man länger anspannen und kürzer entspannen. Aber grundsätzlich soll die Entspannung und die Lockerung des Körpers bei der ganzen Übung im Vordergrund bleiben. Dadurch werden die Muskeln besser trainiert und die Bänder bleiben elastischer.

5. Die Atmung: Bei den Übungen I und IX soll man auf ganz natürliche Art und Weise atmen (zuerst einatmen, dann ausatmen). Bei den Übungen II - VI und VIII wird bei einer Bewegung eingeatmet und bei der nächsten Bewegung ausgeatmet. Bei der Übung VII kann man bei jeder Bewegung einmal ein- und ausatmen. Voraussetzung dafür ist, dass die Übung langsam gemacht wird.

6. Die neun Übungen des „Sehnen- und Knochen-QiGong" können je nach Bedarf einzeln oder komplett geübt werden.

7. Die Trainingsbekleidung sollte weit, locker und weich sein.

8. Nach der Übung die Gelenke warm halten, um sie so vor der Kälte zu schützen. Ebenso nicht zu viel Wasser auf einmal trinken. Besser ist, kleine Mengen auf einen längeren Zeitraum verteilt zu trinken.

9. Bei Fieber und Arthritis sollte man die Übung nicht machen. Wer Rückenschmerzen und Schmerzen an den Beinen, Leber- oder Nierenkrankheiten hat, sollte die Übung vorsichtig ausführen oder vorher den Rat eines Arztes einholen.

# QiGong of the Sinews and Bones (JinGu Gong)

## Introduction

Draw and stretch your sinews, stabilize your bones

The "QiGong of the Sinews and Bones" is a kind of sport using systematic movement of the entire body. It is a special concept for adults and the elderly. Its aim is to slow down the ageing process, to lengthen the duration of life and to improve independence in everyday life. Sinews and bones are like twins. They complete each other, they are interdependent and they exist in unison. Thanks to the functional coordination of sinews, bones and muscles, all activities of the human body (movements) can be performed.

The sinews ought to be stretched, tight and elastic. The bones ought to be solid, strong and tough and must be able to resist pressure. The movements in the joints should be flexible and in carrying them out pliable and smooth. Young people should have hardly any difficulties to meet the requirements quoted above. But in the process of natural ageing, the sinews slowly shrink, the bones grow breakable and brittle. The movability of the joints is more and more impeded, blocked and hindered. Many older people have their backs bowed, their legs and hands have no more power, when walking they are unstable and shaky, and they have difficulties in straightening their bodies and their limbs. To overcome these problems of health you not only must know the causes of the illnesses, but you have got to overcome the blockings actively and bodily. According to Traditional Chinese Medicine Qi (energy) and the blood are circulating fluently as soon as the bones are strong and the sinews are supple. When the energy and blood channels are free, the body does not feel any pain. A well - known quotation from the "Canon of Internal Medicine" (NeiJing)[1] runs: To lengthen the sinews by one Cun[2] means to win ten years of life. This is why it is very important to stretch now and again, to strengthen the bones and to train the pliability and suppleness of the body.

When training the "QiGong of the Sinews and Bones" you have to get used to the exercises step by step. The exercises prove to be especially effective if you carry them out continually over a length of time.

Professor Ding HongYu    NanJing, 15th May 2012

[1] The NeiJing is a collection of 81 lessons that are summed up in two parts. As a medical work it is fundamental and leading in the study of Traditional Chinese Medicine to this very day.

[2] The Cun is a traditional Chinese measure. One Cun has 3,33 centimetres.

## Important Points for the Exercise

1. Before starting the exercise mobilize your muscles and ligaments by means of adequate light preparing exercises. Then warm up your body with the help of quicker and more intensive movements in order to sweat lightly.

2. The intensity, measure of extension and the velocity of the exercise have got to be individually defined and regulated, likewise the frequency of the repetitions. Everybody must be aware of his personal bodily limits.

3. You can start exercising the "QiGong of Sinews and Bones" at any time. In order to make some progress the exercise should be carried out three times a week for 20 to 30 minutes. You can carry out the exercise daily, integrating it into your everyday routine.

4. Tension and relaxing should be combined well in the exercise. Sometimes you should tense for a longer time and relax for a shorter span. Fundamentally, the process of relaxing and loosening of the body should be foremost in the entire exercise. In this way the muscels are trained better and the ligaments stay more elastic.

5. Breathing: In exercises I and IX you should breathe completely naturally (first breathing in, then breathing out). In exercises II - VI and VIII you breathe in while you fulfill one movement and breathe out with the next movement. In exercise VII you can breathe in and out once during each movement. Condition here is that you do the exercise slowly.

6. The nine exercises of the "QiGong of Sinews and Bones" can be carried out singly or completely as occasion demands.

7. Your training dress should be loose and soft.

8. After the exercise keep your joints warm in order to protect them from cold. Moreover, you should not drink too much water at a time. It is better to drink small quantities during a longer span of time.

9. In case of fever or arthritis you should not carry out the exercise. Everybody feeling a pain in the back or in the legs or persons with illnesses of the liver or kidney should carry out the exercise cautiously or should consult a doctor of medicine before starting.

## 标记注释

a）箭头指出运动方向，用左手臂和左腿做的动作用间断的线条表示，用右手臂和右腿做的动作用不间断的线条表示。用点连成的线条指出头部和腰部的转动方向。箭头结束的地方同时也是下一个动作的开始。重复动作的开始用红色箭头标示。

b）在圆圈内的数字标示动作第几节。它和框架一样，也表示动作段落结束，既一个动作的结束和下一个动作的开始。

a）

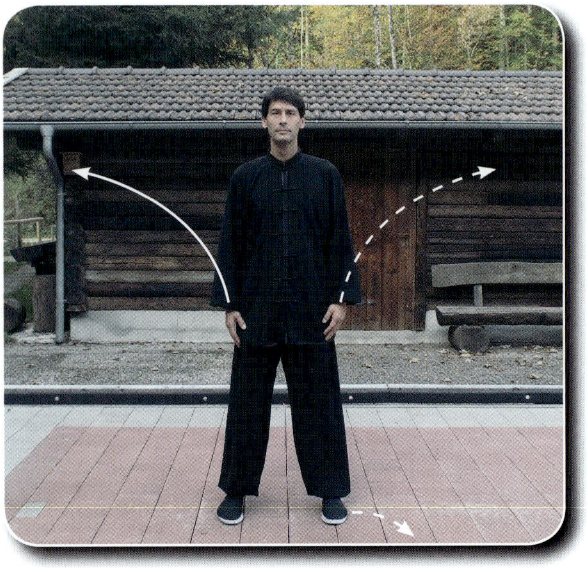

左箭头
links
left

右箭头
rechts
right

头部和腰部的方向
Kopf-/Hüftrichtung
head/hip direction

重复
Wiederholung
repetition

## Zeichenerklärungen

a) Die Pfeile geben die Bewegungsrichtungen vor. Die Bewegungen mit dem linken Arm und dem linken Bein sind mit einer gestrichelten Linie dargestellt, die Bewegungen mit rechts mit einer durchgezogenen Linie.
Die Bewegungen des Kopfes und der Hüfte bzw. Taille werden mit einer gepunkteten Linie dargestellt. Das Ende der Pfeilspitze ist immer die Anfangsposition der darauffolgenden Bewegung. Der Anfang einer Wiederholung ist mit roten Pfeilen gekennzeichnet.
b) Die Zahl im Kreis gibt den Bewegungsabschnitt der jeweiligen Übung an. Außerdem zeigt sie, ebenso wie der Rahmen, das Ende eines Bewegungsabschnitts.

## Key to the Symbols Used

a) The arrows show the directions of movement. The movements with the left arm and the left leg are symbolized by a broken line, the movements on the right hand side with an unbroken line.
The movements of the head and the hip and waist respectively are shown with a dotted line. The end of the arrow point always marks the initial position of the following movement. The beginning of a repetition is marked by red arrows.
b) The number in the circle shows the sequence of movement in each exercise. Apart from this the number shows – like the frame – the end of each sequence of movement.

b)

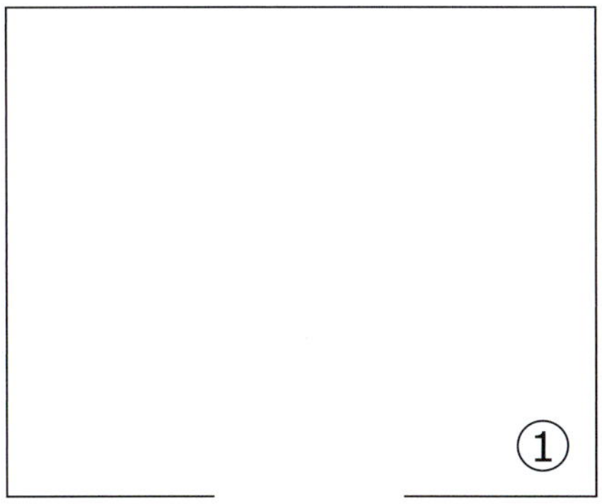


动作段落结束
Ende des Bewegungsabschnitts
end of sequence of movement

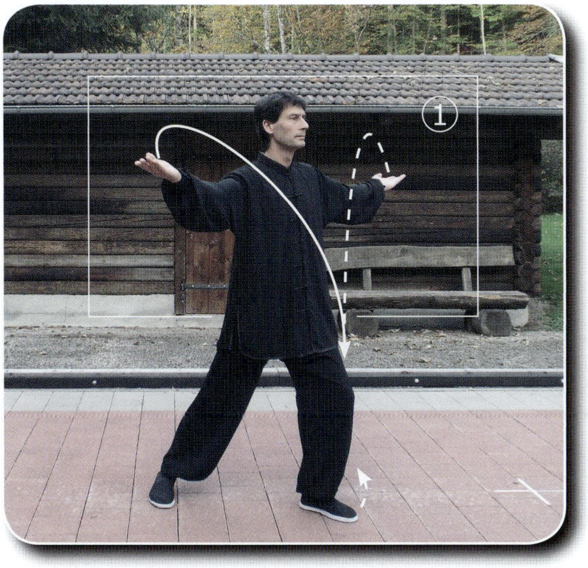

## 练习动作

一、太公行书

二、多面推掌

三、握拳下蹲

四、展臂舒胸

五、拙童脱衣

六、震撼大地

七、寿星练武

八、孔雀开屏

九、踏步展掌

## Die Übungen

I. Der alte Herr übt Kalligraphie (TaiGong XingShu)

II. Die Handflächen in mehrere Richtungen schieben

III. Fäuste machen und die Knie beugen

IV. Die Arme öffnen und die Brust herausstrecken

V. Ein unbeholfenes Kind zieht seine Kleidung aus

VI. Die Erde schütteln

VII. Der Gott der Langlebigkeit praktiziert die Kampfkunst

VIII. Der Pfau öffnet seine Flügel und schlägt das Rad

IX. Auf der Stelle treten und die Hände öffnen

## The Exercises

I. The Old Gentleman Practises Calligraphy (TaiGong XingShu)

II. Shove Your Palms into Several Directions

III. Make Fists and Bend Your Knees

IV. Open Your Arms and Spread Your Chest

V. A Clumsy Child Takes off Its Garments

VI. Shake the Ground

VII. The God of Longevity Practises Martial Art

VIII. The Peacock Opens Its Wings and Spreads Its Tail

IX. Step at the Same Spot and Open Your Hands

预备姿势：两脚开立，与肩同宽，双手垂于体侧，气沉丹田，目光平视，呼吸自然，全身放松。（图1）

## 一、太公行书 8 × 2

两手叉腰（四指在前）。（图2）

第一个8拍：
1—6、用下巴正写‘米’字，6拍完成。（图3）
7—8、再用下巴绕米字以顺时针划大圆一周，两拍完成。（图4）

第二个8拍同第一个8拍。用下巴反写‘米’字，唯有左右方向相反。

整个动作要求头颈动，而身不动，幅度以大为佳。意守“大椎穴”。

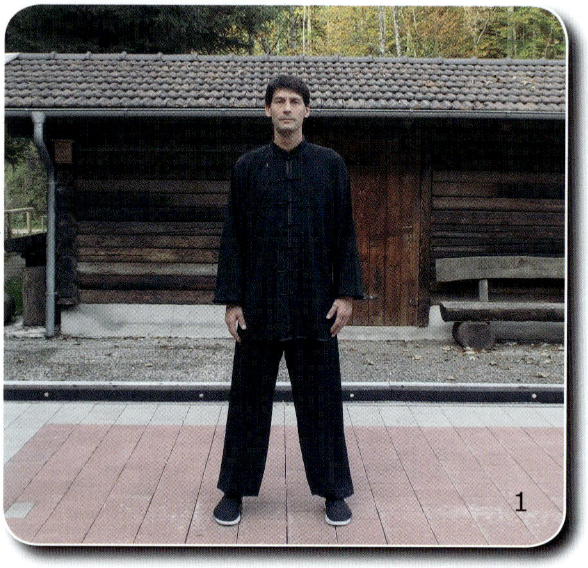
1

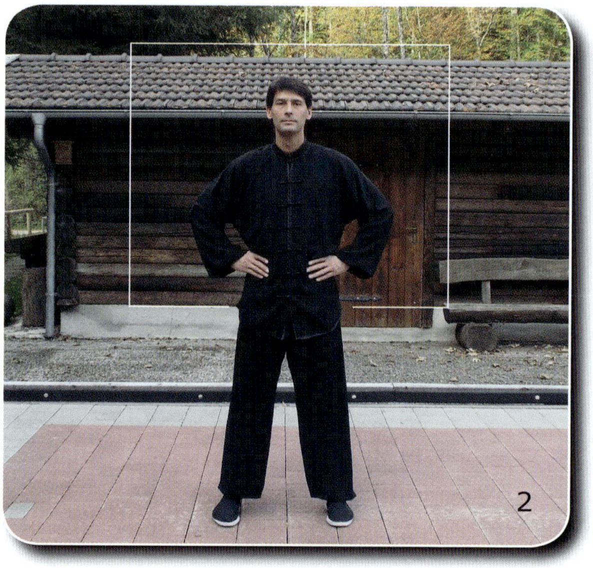
2

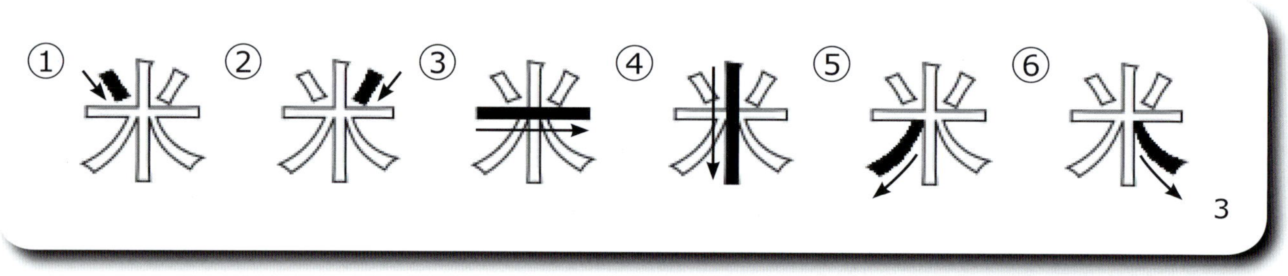

3

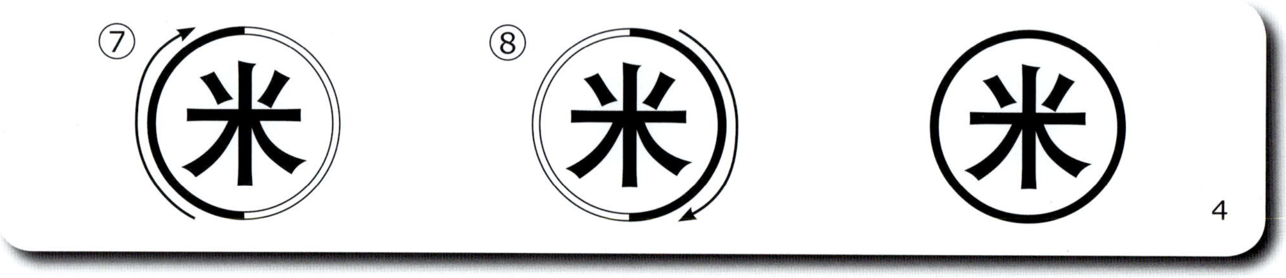

4

Ausgangsstellung: Die Füße parallel stellen, schulterbreit auseinander. Die Arme hängen an den Seiten des Körpers. Qi (Energie) sinkt in das DanTian (Energiezentrum). Den Blick nach vorne richten. Natürlich atmen und den ganzen Körper entspannen. Siehe Bild 1.

## I. Der alte Herr übt Kalligraphie (TaiGong XingShu)

Die Hände zu den Hüften bringen (Finger nach vorne, Daumen nach hinten). Siehe Bild 2.

1. — 6. Mit dem Kinn das Wort Mi (Reis) '米' schreiben. Das Zeichen wird im Stil der Kursivschrift der chinesischen Kalligraphie geschrieben. Die Striche werden gleichsam von links oben zur Mitte (1), von rechts oben zur Mitte (2), dann von links nach rechts (3), von oben nach unten (4), von der Mitte nach links unten (5) und von der Mitte nach rechts unten (6) geschrieben. Siehe Bild 3.
7. — 8. Mit dem Kinn einen großen Kreis um das Wort Mi in Richtung des Uhrzeigers schreiben. Siehe Bild 4.
Die gleichen Bewegungen 1 — 8 nun seitenverkehrt ausführen.

Anforderungen: Nur den Kopf bewegen, nicht den Körper. Die Kopfbewegung soll möglichst groß sein. Die Vorstellungskraft wird auf den Punkt DaZhui gerichtet (YiShou DaZhui).

Initial position: Put your feet parallel, a shoulder breadth apart from each other. Your arms dangle at the sides of your body. Your Qi (energy) sinks into DanTian (centre of energy). Direct your view in front of yourself. Breathe naturally und relax your entire body. See illustration 1.

## I. The Old Gentleman Practises Calligraphy (TaiGong XingShu)

Guide your hands to your hips (your fingers to the front and your thumbs towards the back). See illustration 2.

1. — 6. Write the word Mi (rice) '米' with your chin. The sign is written in the style of the italicised writing of Chinese calligraphy. The "strokes" are written from the left hand upper side to the middle (1), from the right hand upper side to the middle (2), then from left to right (3), from up above downwards (4), from the middle down to the left hand side (5) and from the middle down to the right hand side (6). See illustration 3.
7. — 8. Write a big circle with your chin around the word Mi in the direction of the hands of the clock. See illustration 4.
Carry out the same movements 1 — 8, but to the other side.

Requirements: Move your head only, not your body. The movement of your head ought to be as expansive as possible. Your mind is directed to DaZhui Point (YiShou DaZhui).

## 二、多面推掌

（前后、左右、上下）立掌推，握拳收。

1、两脚不动，身体左转90度，同时双手分别向体侧推掌，手指朝上。（图1，2）

2、身体转正，两手握拳收于腰间，拳心朝上。（图3）

3—4动同1—2动，其方向相反。(图4，5)

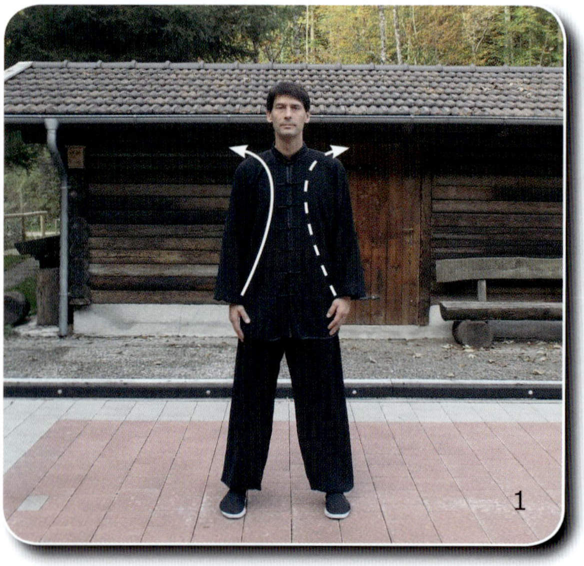


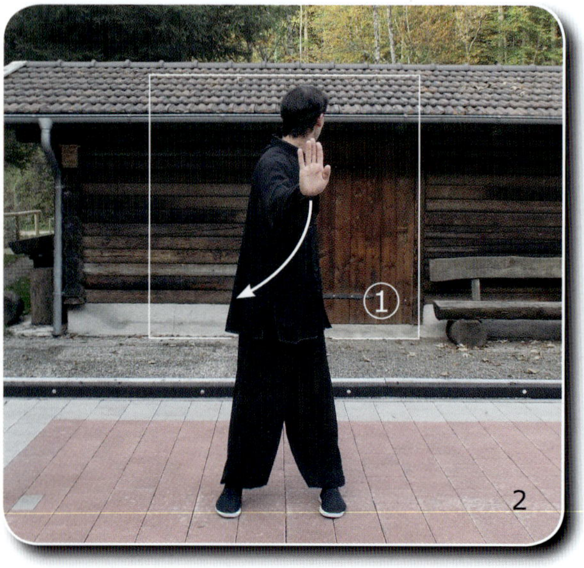


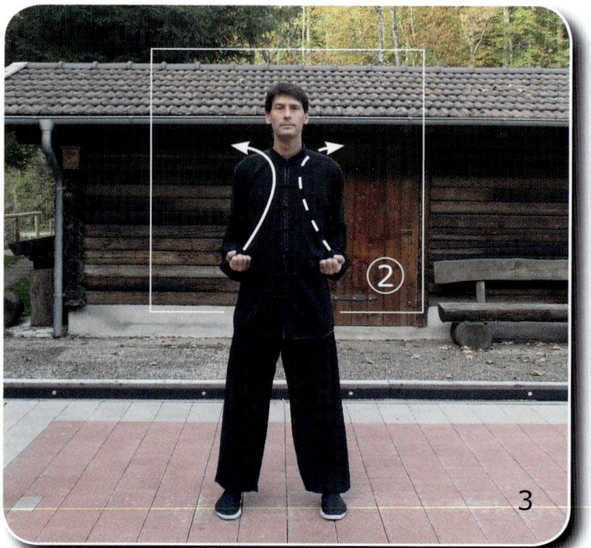

## II. Die Handflächen in mehrere Richtungen schieben

(vorne und hinten, links und rechts, oben und unten)

1. Die Füße nicht bewegen und den Körper um 90° nach links drehen. Dabei gleichzeitig die Arme anheben und die Handflächen zur Seite schieben. Die Handflächen sind aufgerichtet, die Finger zeigen nach oben. Der Blick geht zur linken Hand. Siehe Bilder 1 und 2.
2. Den Körper wieder nach vorne drehen. Die Hände umdrehen, so dass die Handflächen nach oben schauen. Anschließend die Hände zur Faust schließen und zurück zu den Hüften ziehen. Siehe Bild 3.
3. — 4. Die gleichen Bewegungen wie 1 — 2 in die entgegengesetzte Richtung ausführen. Siehe Bilder 4 und 5.

## II. Shove Your Palms into Several Directions

(front and back, left and right, up and down)

1. Do not move your feet and turn your body by 90° to the left. At the same time lift your arms and push both your palms to the side. Your palms are turned upwards, your fingers show upwards. Your view is directed to your left hand. See illustrations 1 and 2.
2. Turn your body to the front side again. Turn your hands so that your palms point upwards. Then close your hands making a fist and guide them back to your hips. See illustration 3.
3. — 4. Carry out the same movements as 1 — 2 in the opposite direction. See illustrations 4 and 5.

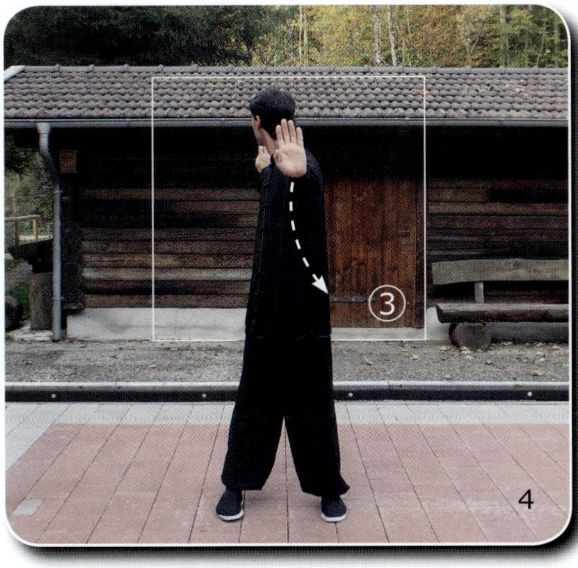


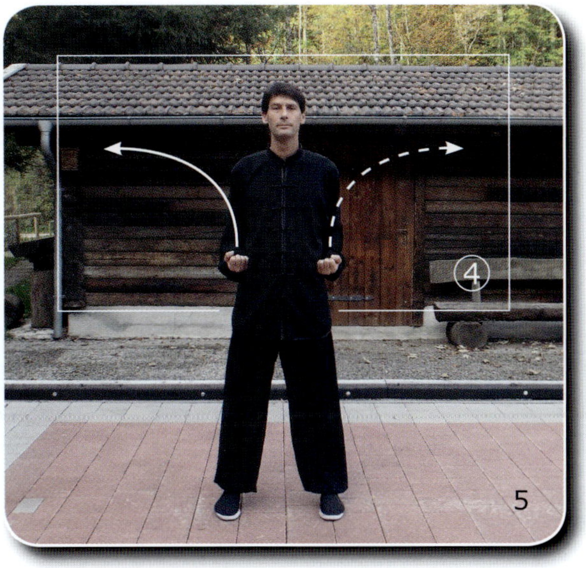

5、双手变掌同时向两侧推出，手指朝上。（图6）
6、两手握拳收于腰间，拳心朝上。 （图7）
7、双手变掌向上推掌，掌心向上，手指向后，两臂与身体尽量成直线。（图8）
8、双手经胸前下按（成预备式）。 （图9，10）

第二个8拍，同第一个8拍。意守劳宫穴 。

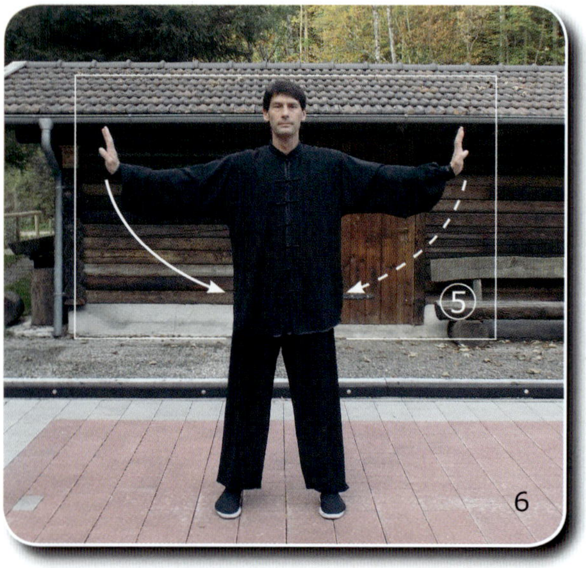


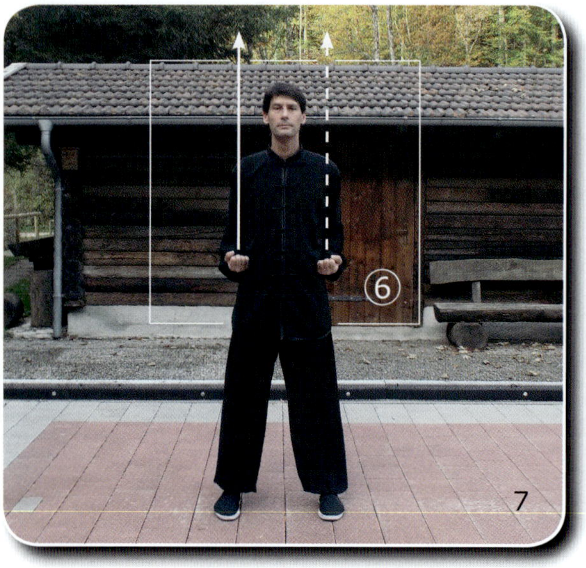


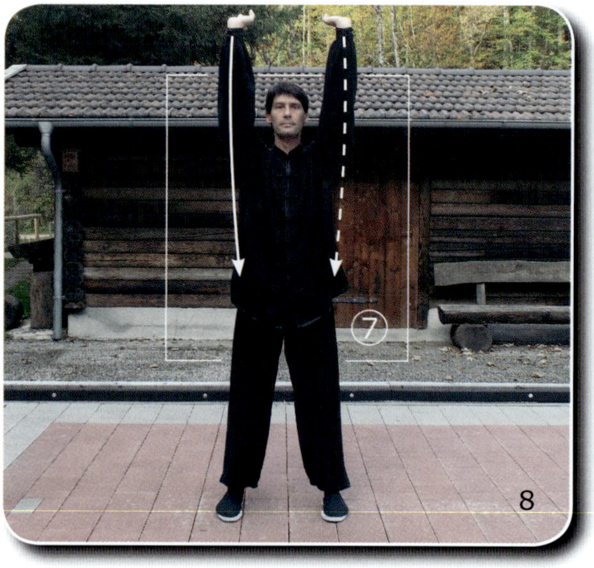

5. Die Fäuste öffnen und die Handflächen zu den Seiten schieben. Die Handflächen sind aufgerichtet, die Finger zeigen nach oben. Siehe Bild 6.
6. Die Hände umdrehen, so dass die Handflächen nach oben schauen. Anschließend die Hände zur Faust schließen und zurück zu den Hüften ziehen. Siehe Bild 7.
7. Die Fäuste öffnen und die Handflächen nach oben schieben. Die Handflächen zeigen nach oben und die Finger nach hinten. Beide Arme parallel ganz gerade zum Körper ausrichten. Siehe Bild 8.
8. Die Handflächen vor der Brust nach unten drücken (zur Ausgangsposition). Siehe Bilder 9 und 10.

Die Bewegungen 1 — 8 ein zweites Mal ausführen. Die Vorstellungskraft wird auf den Punkt LaoGong gerichtet (YiShou LaoGong).

5. Open your fists and push your palms to the sides. Your palms are erect, your fingers pointing upwards. See illustration 6.
6. Turn your hands round so that your palms point upwards. Then close your hands making a fist and drawing them back towards your hips. See illustration 7.
7. Open your fists and push your palms upwards. Your palms point upwards and your fingers to the back. Align both your arms absolutely straightly, parallel to your body. See illustration 8.
8. Push your palms down in front of your chest (to the initial position). See ill. 9 and 10.

The movements 1 — 8 are carried out a second time. Your mind is directed to LaoGong Point (YiShou LaoGong).

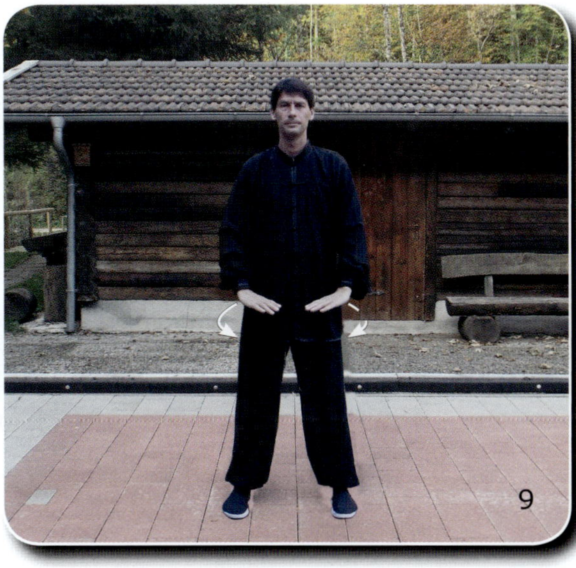
9

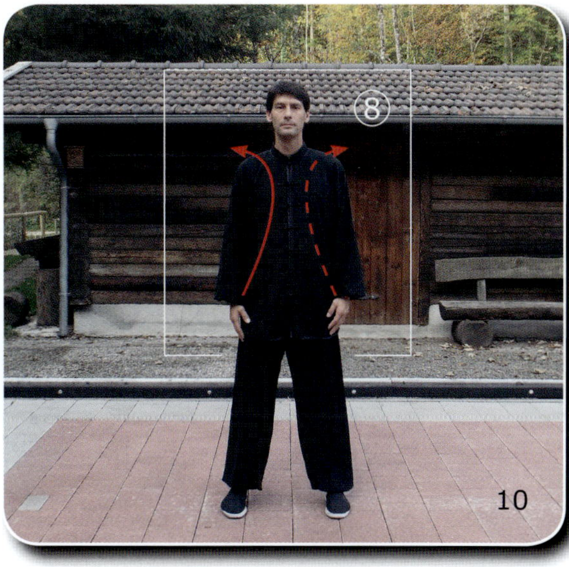

10

## 三、握拳下蹲

第一个8拍:

1、双手前伸, 手指张开（手心向前）， 同时两脚脚趾尖翘起张开。（图1, 2）

2、双手握拳下拉至腰侧， 拳心向下， 中指扣劳宫。同时两腿下蹲十趾抓地。（图3）

3—4动同1—2动。（图4, 5）

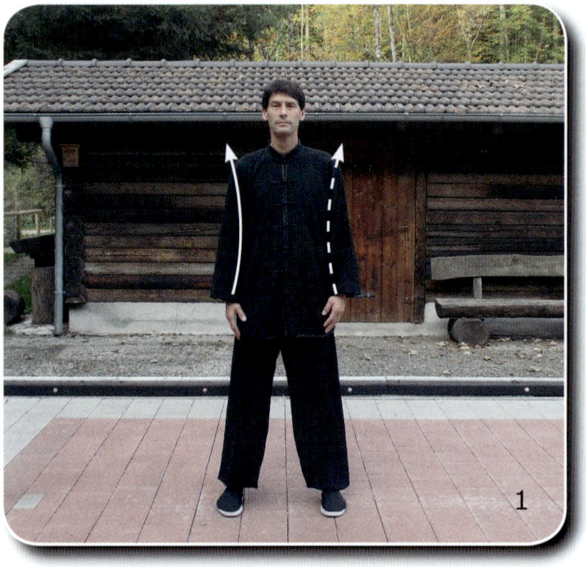
1

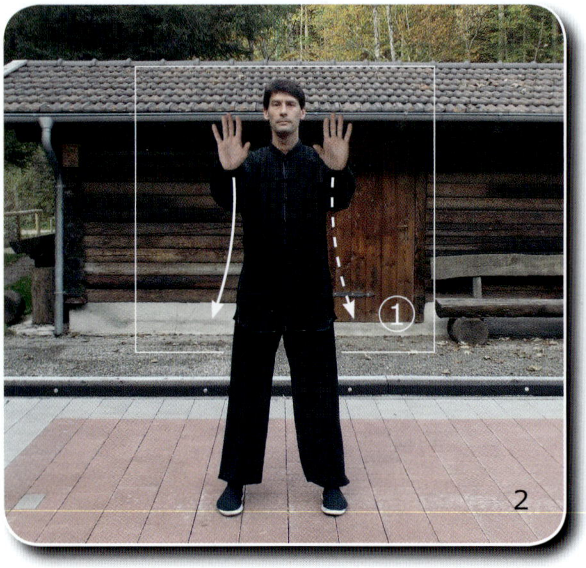

2

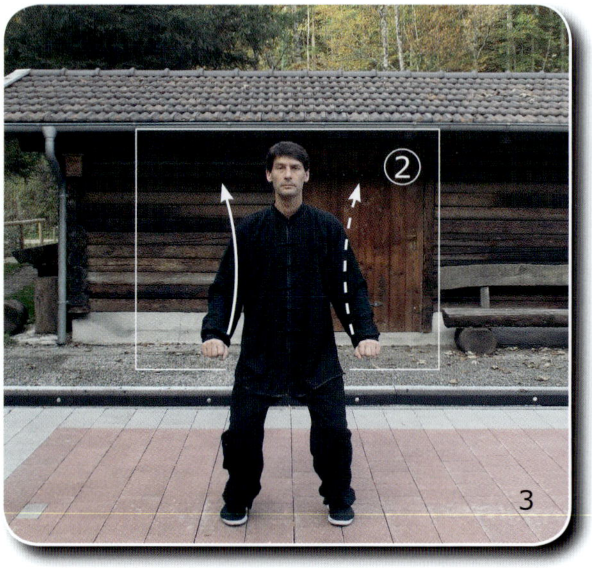

3

## III. Fäuste machen und die Knie beugen

1. Die Hände bis auf Brusthöhe heben und die Handflächen nach vorne schieben. Die Finger sind dabei geöffnet. Gleichzeitig die Zehenspitzen nach oben ziehen und die Zehen spreizen. Siehe Bilder 1 und 2.
2. Beide Hände (Handflächen schauen nach unten) zur Faust schließen und sie nach unten ziehen bis zur Hüfte. Der Mittelfinger drückt auf den Punkt LaoGong. Gleichzeitig die Knie beugen und mit den Zehenspitzen den Boden greifen. Siehe Bild 3.
3. — 4. Die gleichen Bewegungen wie 1 — 2 werden wiederholt. Siehe Bilder 4 und 5.

## III. Make Fists and Bend Your Knees

1. Lift your hands up to chest height and shove your palms forward. Your fingers are opened in doing so. At the same time draw the tips of your toes upwards and spread your toes wide. See illustrations 1 and 2.
2. Close both your hands (palms upwards) into a fist and guide them down to your hips. Your middlefinger presses LaoGong Point. At the same time bend your knees and grip the earth with the tips of your toes. See illustration 3.
3. — 4. The same movements as 1 — 2 are repeated. See illustrations 4 and 5.

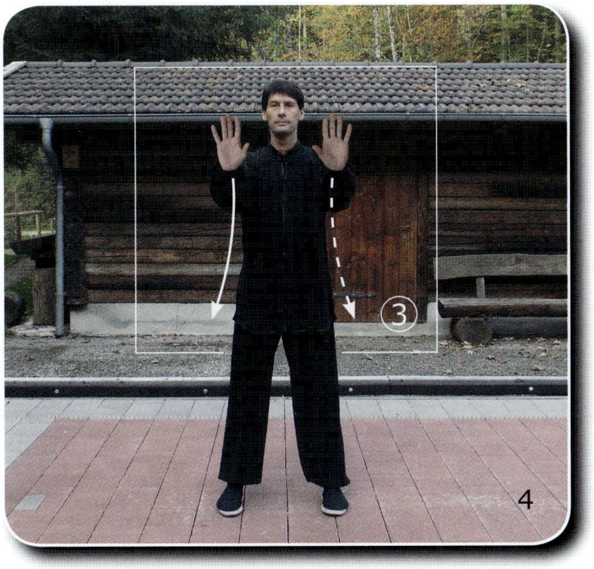

4

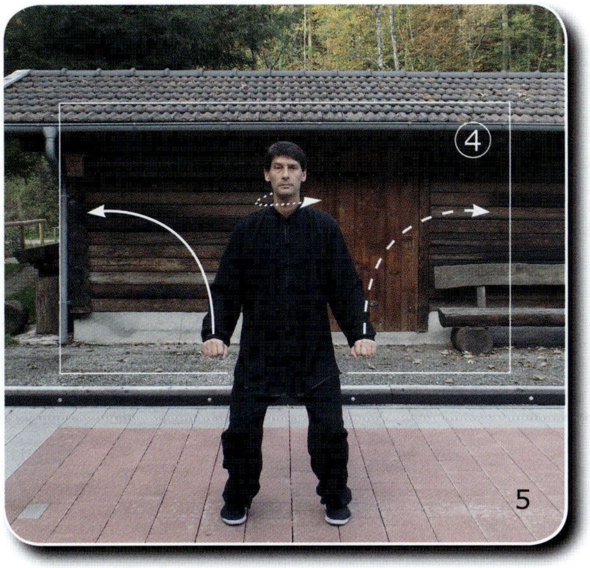

5

5、双手侧伸，手指张开（手心向外），两腿伸直，趾尖翘起张开。（图6）
6、双手握拳下拉至胯侧，拳心向下，中指扣劳宫。同时两腿下蹲十趾抓地。（图7）
7—8动同5—6动，其方向相反。（图8, 9）

第二个8拍同第一个8拍。最后一拍成预备式。本节动作，抓握时要求意守劳宫穴、下蹲时意守涌泉穴。（图10）

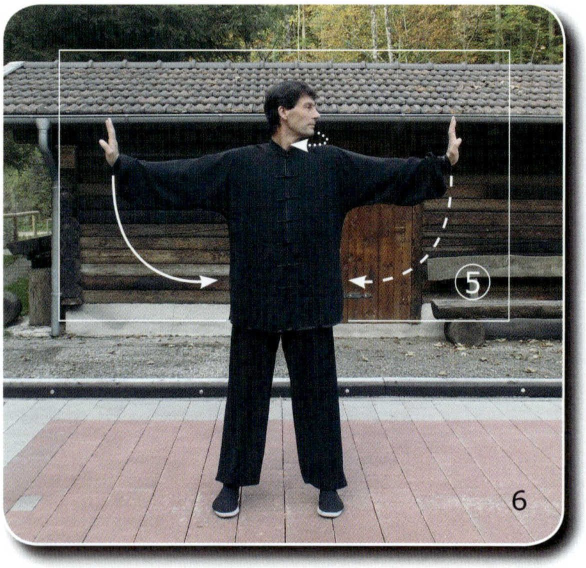

6

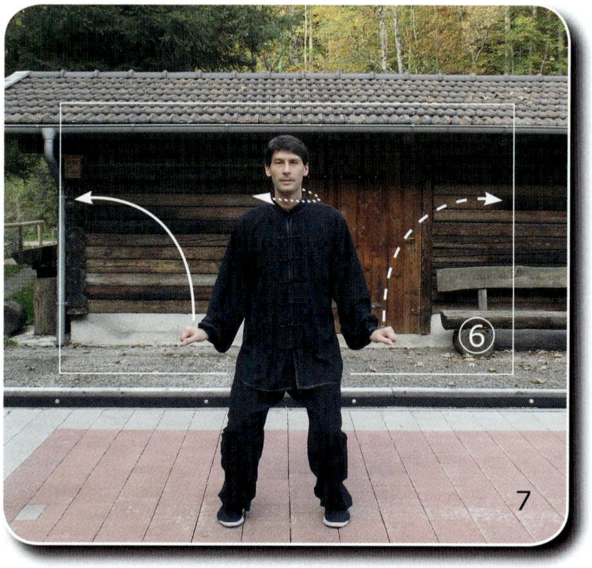

7

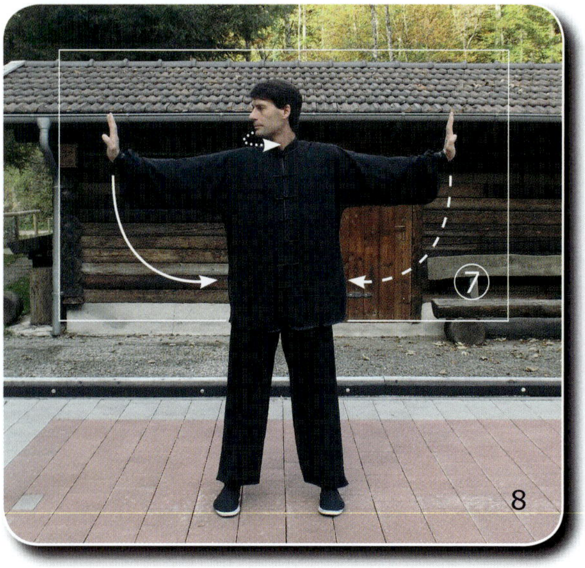

8

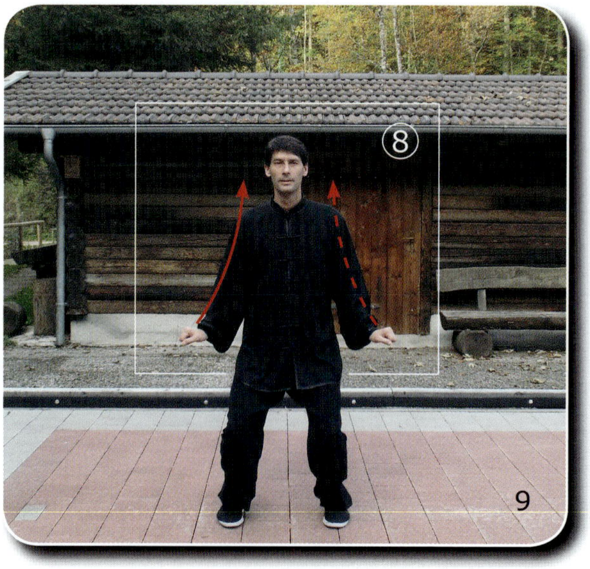

9

5. Die Hände an den Seiten nach oben führen und die Beine wieder gerade machen. Den Kopf nach links drehen und dabei die Handflächen nach außen schieben, die Finger geöffnet. Gleichzeitig die Zehenspitzen nach oben ziehen und spreizen. Siehe Bild 6.
6. Beide Hände (Handflächen schauen nach unten) zur Faust schließen und nach unten ziehen bis zur Hüfte. Der Mittelfinger drückt auf den Punkt LaoGong. Gleichzeitig die Knie beugen und mit den Zehenspitzen den Boden greifen. Den Kopf dabei wieder nach vorne drehen. Bild 7.
7. — 8. Die gleichen Bewegungen wie 5 — 6 zur anderen Seite ausführen. Siehe Bilder 8 und 9.

Die Bewegungen 1 — 8 ein zweites Mal wiederholen. Am Ende des zweiten Durchgangs wieder zurück in die Ausgangsposition gehen (d.h. nur die Fäuste zur Hüfte ziehen ohne die Knie dabei zu beugen). Siehe Bild 10. Die Vorstellungskraft wird beim Zurückziehen der Fäuste auf den Punkt LaoGong (YiShou LaoGong) und beim Beugen der Knie auf den Punkt YongQuan (YiShou YongQuan) gerichtet.

5. Guide your hands upwards at your sides and straighten your legs again. Turn your head to the left and at the same time shove your palms outwards, your fingers opened. Draw the tips of your toes upwards, spread them wide at the same time. See illustration 6.
6. Close both your hands (your palms pointing downwards) into fists and draw them downwards to your hips. Your middlefinger presses the LaoGong Point. At the same time bend your knees and grip the earth with the tips of your toes. Turn your head to the front again. See ill. 7.
7. — 8. Carry out the same movements as 5 — 6 to the other side. See illustrations 8 and 9.

Repeat the movements 1 — 8 a second time. At the end of the second sequence go back to the initial position (i.e. draw your fists only towards your hips without bending your knees). See illustration 10. Your imagination is directed to LaoGong Point (YiShou LaoGong) while drawing back your fists and to YongQuan Point (YiShou YongQuan) while bending your knees.

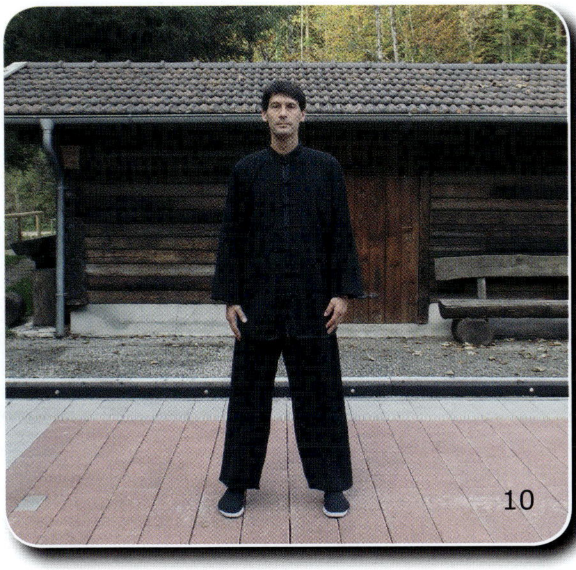
10

## 四、展臂舒胸

1、左脚向前45度方向上步成左弓步，双手经胸前摆至侧平举，掌心向上。（图1，2）
2、体重后移，右腿屈膝支撑，左脚伸直，足尖翘起。同时屈身前俯，双手向上划弧压于左膝上。（图3）
3、身体直起，重心前移于左足，右足尖点地，同时双手上举，手心斜对（成10点10分位置）。（图4）

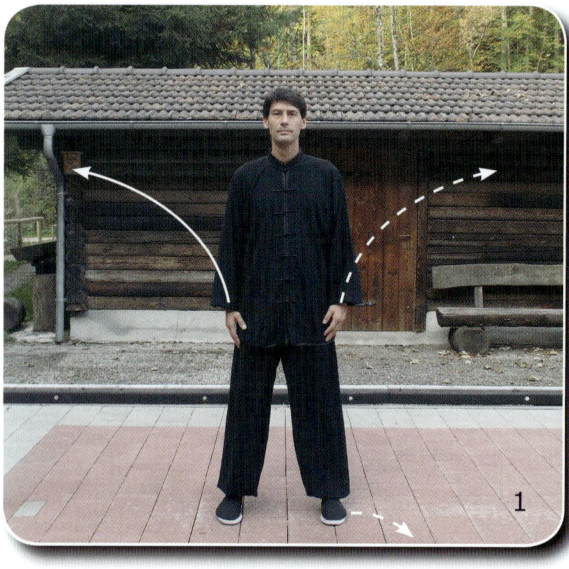


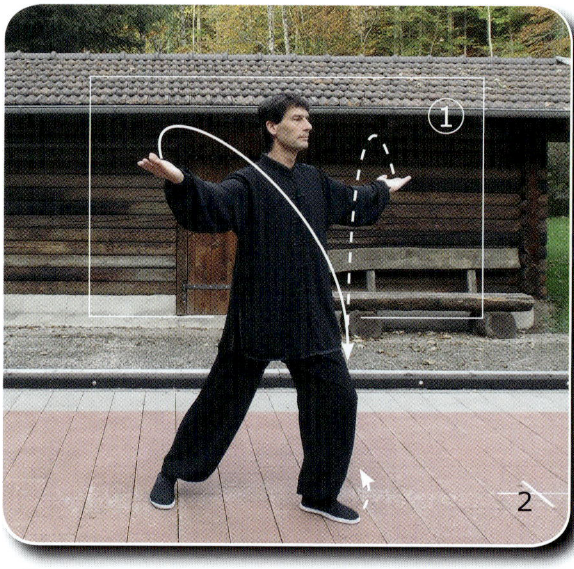


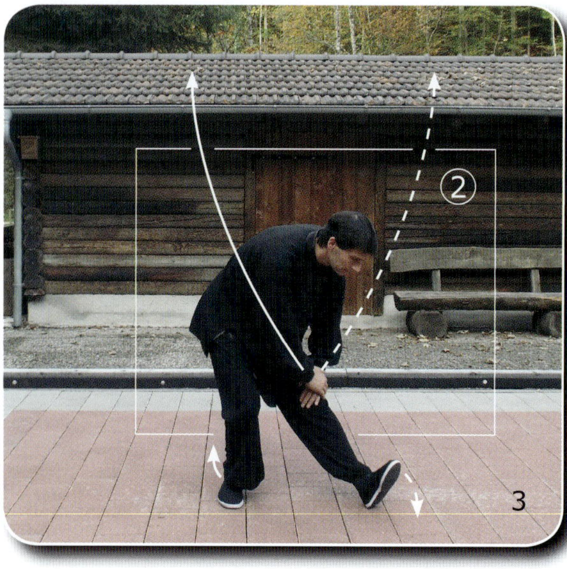


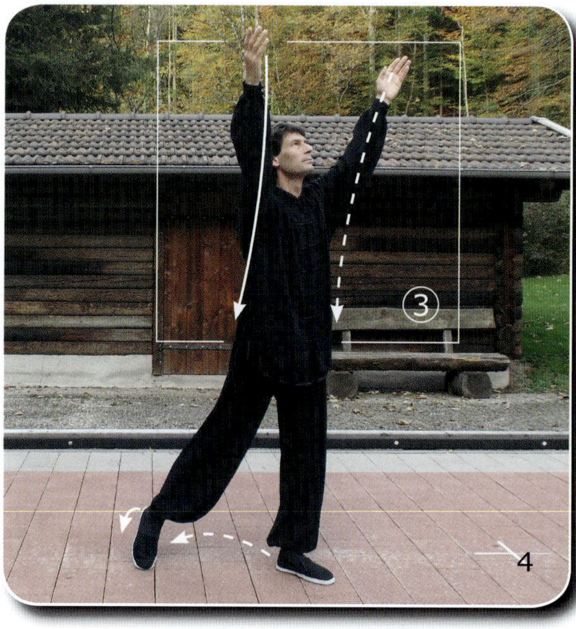

## IV. Die Arme öffnen und die Brust herausstrecken

1. Den linken Fuß etwa 45° nach vorne setzen zu einem GongBu (Bogenschritt). Die Arme vor der Brust auf Schulterhöhe bringen und zur Seite strecken. Die Händflächen schauen nach oben. Siehe Bilder 1 und 2.
2. Das Körpergewicht nach hinten verlagern, das rechte Bein gebeugt, das linke Bein gerade gestreckt. Die Zehen des linken Fußes vom Boden lösen und nach oben strecken. Gleichzeitig den Körper nach vorne beugen, beide Hände in einem Bogen nach unten zum linken Knie führen und darauf drücken. Siehe Bild 3.
3. Den Körper aufrichten, den Schwerpunkt nach vorne auf den linken Fuß verlagern. Dabei die rechte Ferse vom Boden lösen, gleichzeitig die Hände nach oben strecken, die Handflächen schauen zueinander, die Arme sind geöffnet (eine Position wie 10 nach 10 Uhr). Siehe Bild 4.

## IV. Open Your Arms and Spread Your Chest

1. Put your left foot forward about 45° to GongBu Stance (Bowstance). Guide your arms up to shoulder height in front of your chest and spread them to the sides. Your palms point upwards. See illustrations 1 and 2.
2. Shift your body weight backwards, your right leg bent, your left leg straight. Take the toes of your left foot off the ground and stretch them upwards. At the same time bend your body forward, guide both your hands in a bow down to your left knee and press it. See illustration 3.
3. Straighten your body and shift your centre of gravity forward onto your left foot. While doing so take your right heel off the ground and spread your hands upwards at the same time, your palms facing each other, your arms open (a position like the hands of the clock at ten past ten). See illustration 4.

4、身体转正，双手下落，同时左足收回。（图5）
5—8动同1—4动，其方向对称。（图6—9）

共做两个8拍。 最后一拍成预备式。 （图10）
意守丹田。

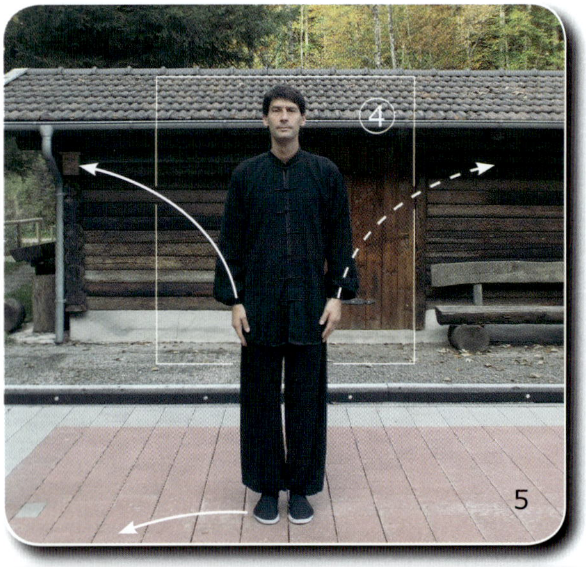

5

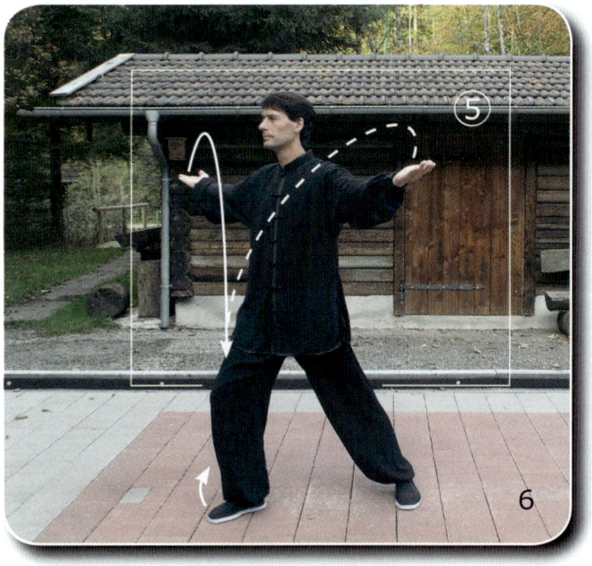

6

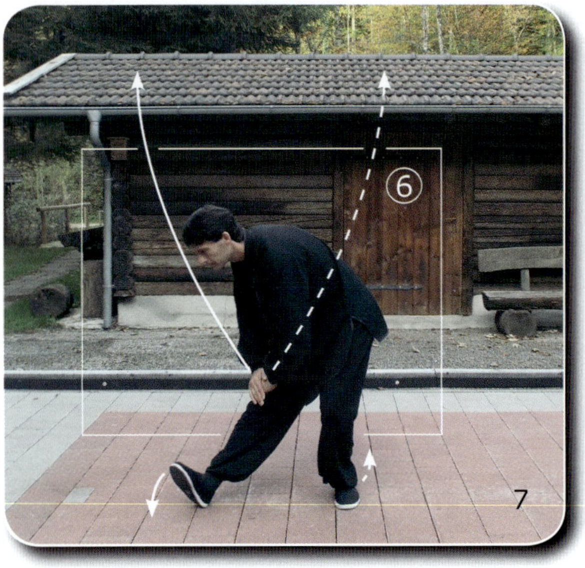

7

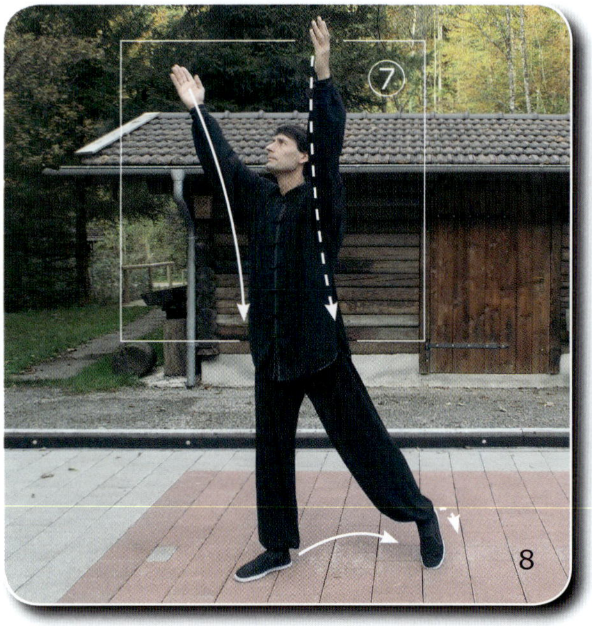

8

4. Den Körper wieder nach vorne ausrichten, beide Hände (Handflächen schauen zueinander) zu den Seiten nach unten bringen. Gleichzeitig das Körpergewicht auf das rechte Bein verlagern und den linken Fuß heransetzen. Siehe Bild 5.
5. — 8. Die gleichen Bewegungen 1 — 4 zur anderen Seite ausführen. Siehe Bilder 6 - 9.

Die Bewegungen 1 — 8 ein zweites Mal wiederholen. Am Ende des zweiten Durchgangs den linken Fuß wieder zur Ausgangsposition bringen. Siehe Bild 10. Die Vorstellungskraft wird auf das DanTian gerichtet (YiShou DanTian).

4. Align your body to the front again and guide both your hands down to your sides (your palms facing each other). At the same time shift your body weight onto your right leg and draw your left foot towards your right foot. See illustration 5.
5. — 8. Carry out the same movements 1 — 4 to the other side. See illustrations 6 - 9.

Repeat the movements 1 — 8 a second time. At the end of the second sequence guide your left foot back to the initial position. See illustration 10. Your imagination is directed on DanTian (YiShou DanTian).

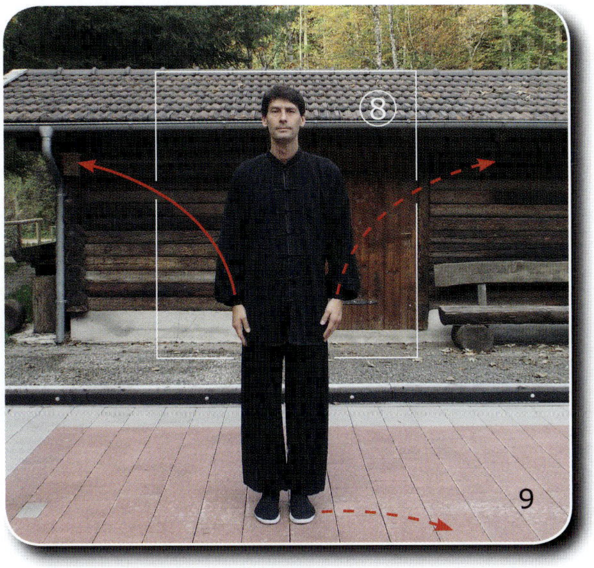

9

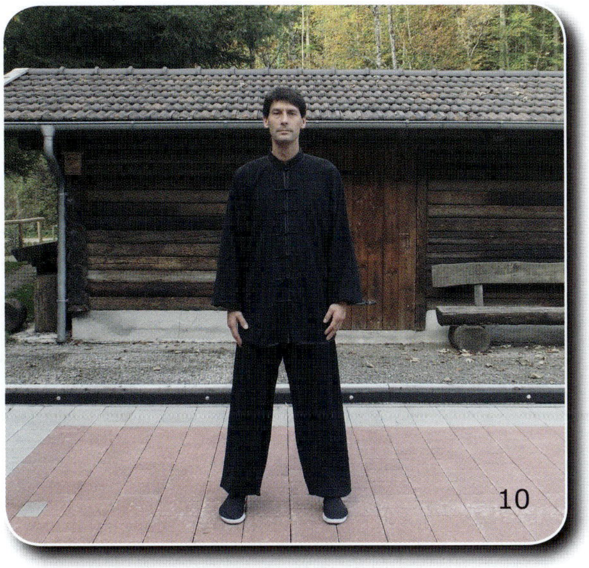
10

## 五、拙童脱衣
（上下疏通）

1、两掌外旋向后上方直臂摆至头顶上方，两掌相合，使身体稍后仰，眼看双手。（图1, 2）
2、两手下行到胸前，转为手指向下，引胃经下行，同时弓身下腰，双手靠近足背。（图3）
3、身体保持不动，两手向前平推。（图4）

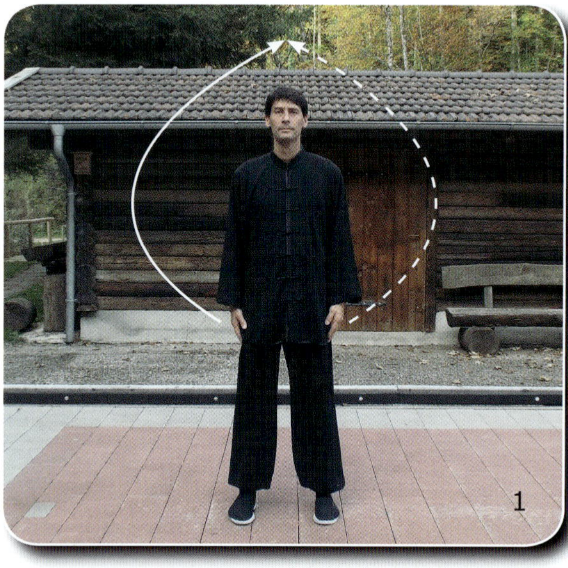
1

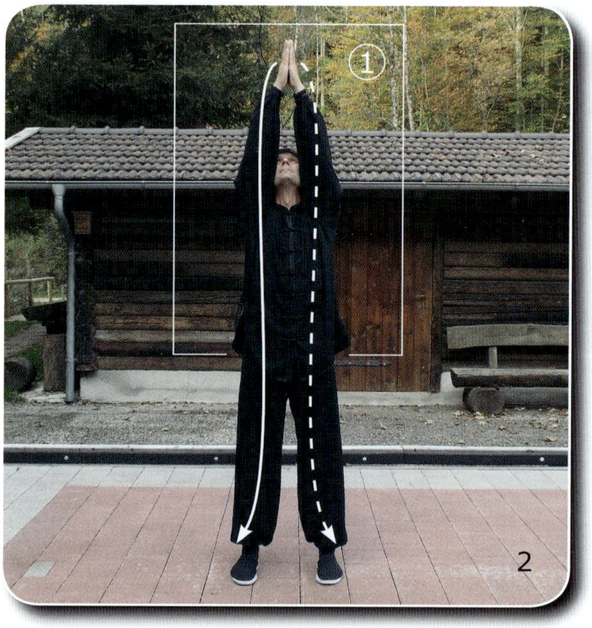

2

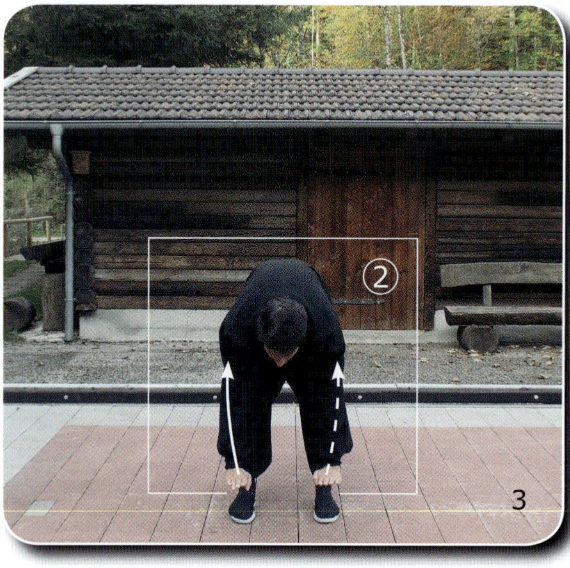

3

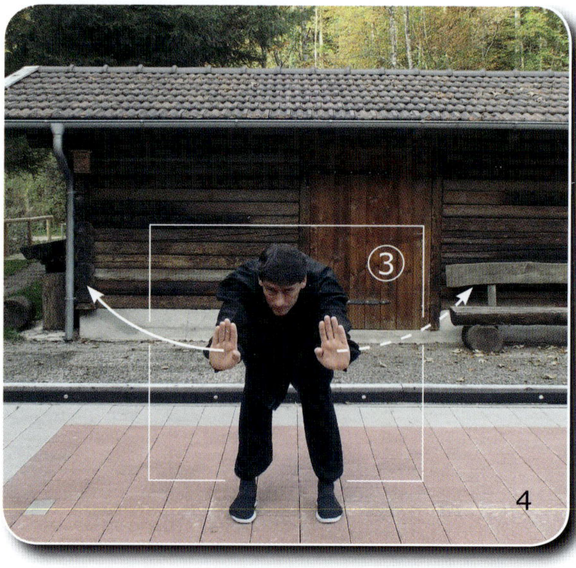

4

## V. Ein unbeholfenes Kind zieht seine Kleidung aus

(Von oben nach unten den Körper durchlässig machen)

1. Die Hände umdrehen (Handflächen schauen nach außen) und die Arme strecken. Dann die Hände nach oben über den Kopf führen, bis sich die Handflächen berühren. Den Körper dabei leicht nach hinten kippen. Der Blick geht nach oben zu den Händen. Siehe Bilder 1 und 2.
2. Die Hände voneinander lösen und nach unten zurück vor die Brust bringen, die Finger zeigen nach unten. Mit den Händen weiter nach unten entlang des WeiJing (Magenmeridians) gleiten. Gleichzeitig den Oberkörper nach unten beugen. Am Ende der Bewegung befinden sich beide Hände (die Finger schauen nach vorne) über den Fußrücken. Siehe Bild 3.
3. Den Körper nicht bewegen, beide Hände flach über den Boden nach vorne schieben. Siehe Bild 4.

## V. A Clumsy Child Takes off Its Garments

(Make your body permeable from up above downwards)

1. Turn your hands (your palms showing outside) and stretch your arms. Then guide your hands upwards above your head until your palms touch each other. While doing so tip your body over slighty to the back. Your view goes upwards to your hands. See illustrations 1 and 2.
2. Disconnect your hands and guide them downwards back in front of your breast, your fingers pointing downwards. Glide further downwards along WeiJing (Meridian of Your Stomach) with your hands. Bend the upper part of your body downwards at the same time. At the end of the movement both your hands are situated above the backs of your feet (your fingers pointing to the front). See illustration 3.
3. Do not move your body and shove your hands to the front flatly above the ground. See illustration 4.

4、双手边回拉边向两侧打开，再交叉于胸前，同时身体略下蹲。（图5, 6）
5、两手沿两腿外侧上行（同时上体抬起）两手经于带脉。（图7）
6、双手继续上行（模仿脱衣）。（图8）
7、两手伸直（与1动相同）。（图9）
8、双手由两侧下落成预备式。（图10）

共做两个8拍。意守命门。

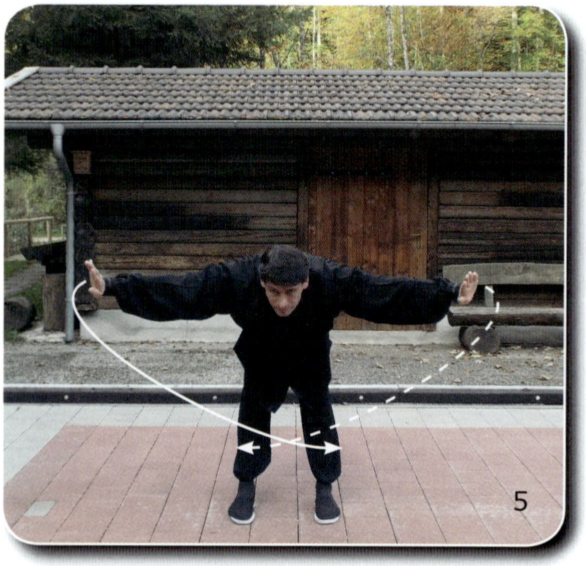


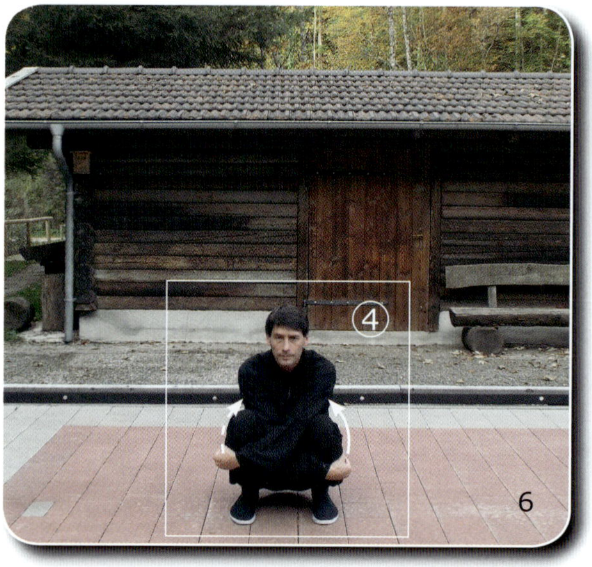


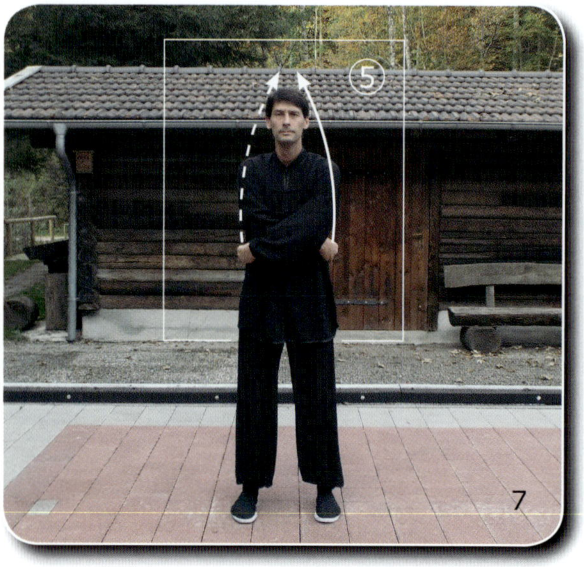


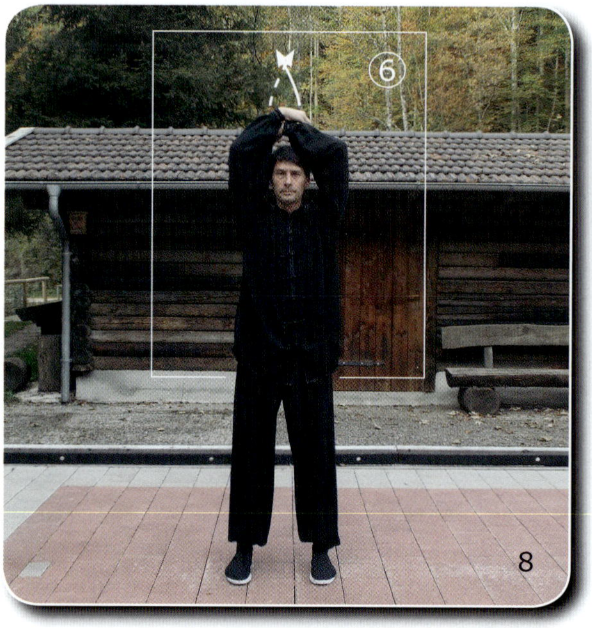

4. Die Hände zur Seite öffnen. Anschließend in die Hocke gehen, dabei die Hände zurückziehen und überkreuzen. Die Hände befinden sich am Ende der Bewegung an den Außenseiten der Unterschenkel. Siehe Bilder 5 und 6.
5. Die Hände an den Außenseiten der Beine nach oben bewegen bis zum Gürtelgefäß (DaiMai), gleichzeitig den Oberkörper aufrichten. Siehe Bild 7.
6. Die Hände weiter nach oben an den Außenseiten des Körpers entlang führen, als ob man sich ausziehen würde. Siehe Bild 8.
7. Die Arme gerade strecken, bis sich die Handflächen wieder berühren. Siehe Bild 9.
8. Die Hände seitlich nach unten bringen zur Ausgangsposition. Siehe Bild 10.

Die Bewegungen 1 — 8 ein zweites Mal wiederholen. Die Vorstellungskraft wird auf den Punkt MingMen gerichtet (YiShou MingMen).

4. Open your hands to the sides. Then squat and in doing so draw your hands back and cross them. At the end of the movement your hands are at the outsides of your shin-bones. See illustrations 5 and 6.
5. Move your hands upwards at the outsides of your legs up to Belt Meridian (DaiMai), at the same time straighten the upper part of your body. See illustration 7.
6. Guide your hands farther upwards along the outsides of your body as if undressing yourself. See illustration 8.
7. Straighten your arms until your palms touch each other again. See illustration 9.
8. Take your hands down at your sides to the initial position. See illustration 10.

Repeat the movements 1 — 8 a second time. Your imagination is directed at MingMen Point (YiShou MingMen).

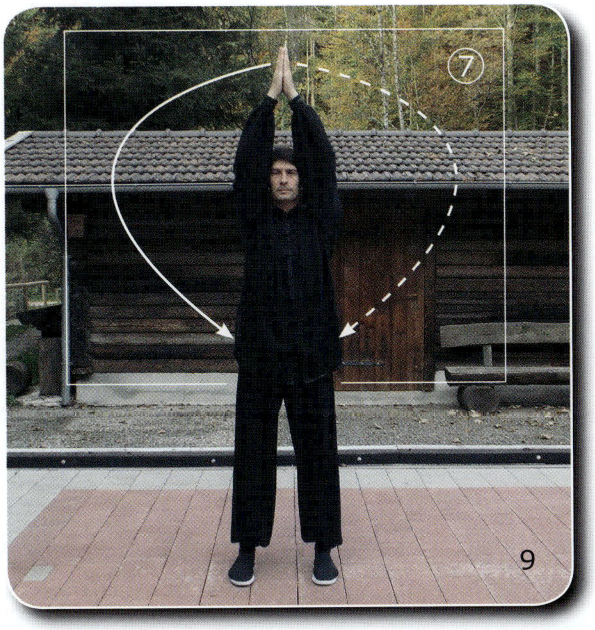


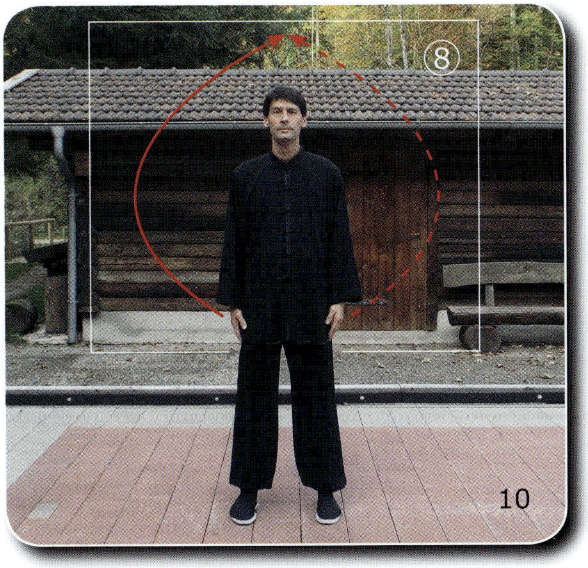

## 六、震撼大地

1、两手握拳经胸前交叉外翻至侧上举，拳心向前。（图1, 2）
2、双拳经两侧用力向下击打‘环跳’，同时双腿半蹲成马步，并大力发出‘嘿！’声。（图3）
3、双手分别向两侧上提成侧平举，（手心向上）同时两腿伸直。（图4）

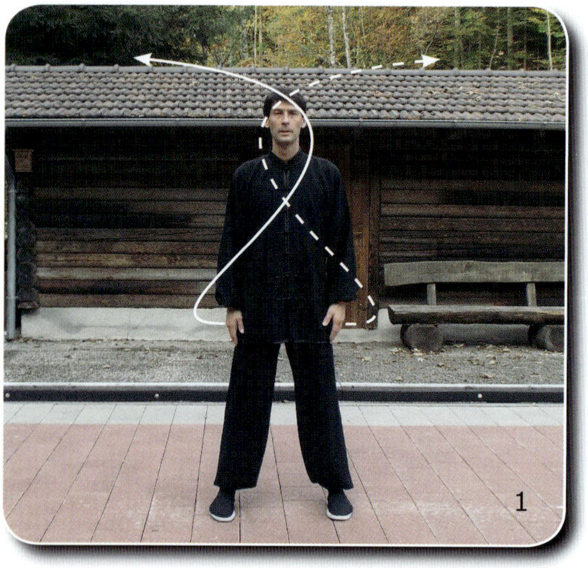


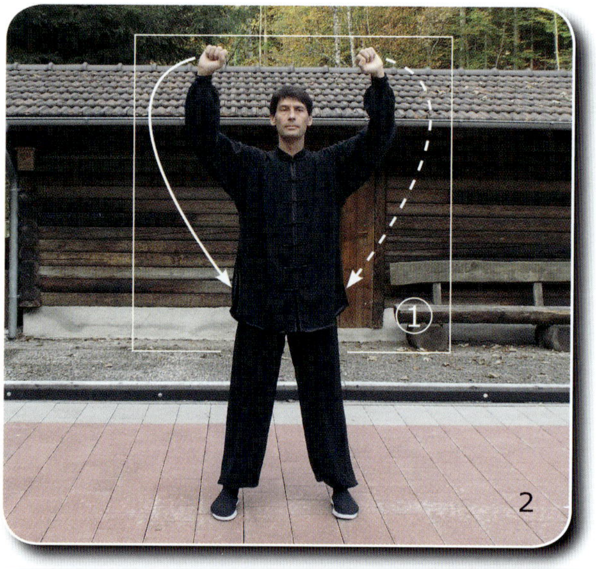


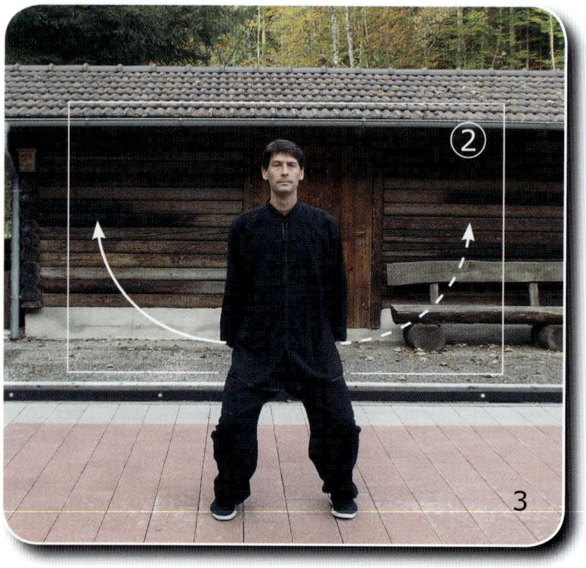


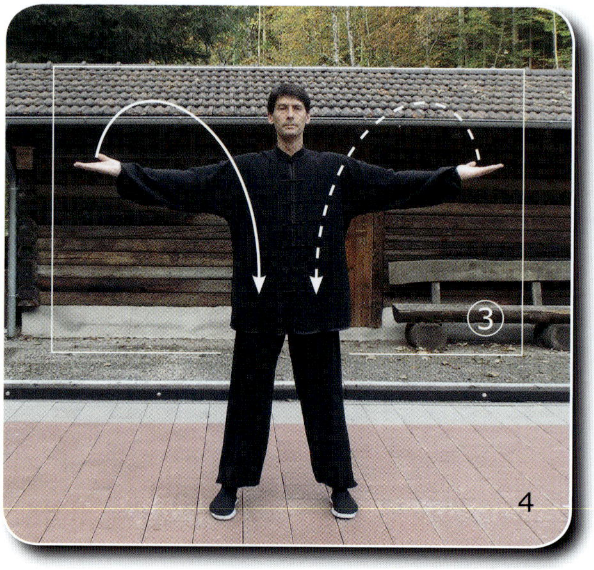

## VI. Die Erde schütteln

1. Die Hände etwas zur Seite bringen (nach links und rechts). Dann die Hände zur Faust schließen und vor der Brust kreuzen (die Handrücken zeigen zur Brust). Anschließend weiter nach oben schieben und auf Stirnhöhe die Kreuzung der Arme lösen, dann die Fäuste zur Seite schieben. Die Handrücken der Fäuste schauen nach hinten. Siehe Bilder 1 und 2.
2. Die Fäuste seitlich nach unten bringen und kräftig auf den Punkt HuanTiao schlagen. Gleichzeitig die Beine beugen zur Stellung des MaBu (Stellung des Pferdes) und den Laut „Hei" von sich geben. Siehe Bild 3.
3. Die Fäuste öffnen und die Hände seitlich anheben bis zur Waagerechten in Schulterhöhe, die Handflächen schauen nach oben. Gleichzeitig die Beine gerade strecken. Siehe Bild 4.

## VI. Shake the Ground

1. Guide your hands somewhat to your sides (left and right). Then close your hands into fists and cross them in front of your chest (the backs of your hands pointing towards your chest). Next push them upwards and undo the crossing of your arms at the height of your forehead, then push your fists to the sides. The backs of your fists point backwards. See illustrations 1 and 2.
2. Take your fists down at the sides and beat at HuanTiao Point powerfully. At the same time bend your legs to the Postion of MaBu (Position of the Horse) and utter the sound "Hei". See illustration 3.
3. Open your fists and raise your hands at the sides up to horizontal position at shoulder height, your palms pointing upwards. At the same time straighten your legs. See illustration 4.

4、两手经胸前成马步按掌，两手指尖相对。（图5）
5—8动同1—4动。共做两个8拍。（图6—9）

最后一拍成预备式。（图10）
意守涌泉穴。

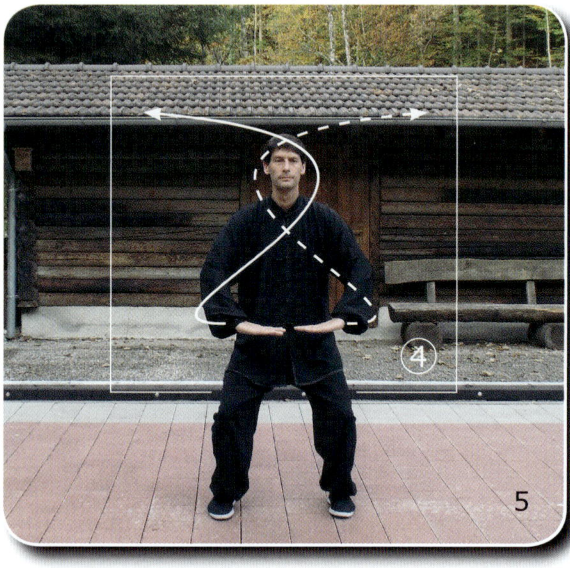

5

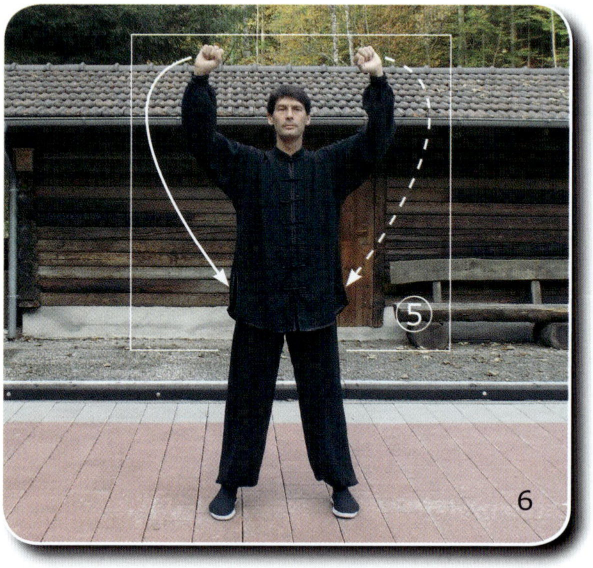

6

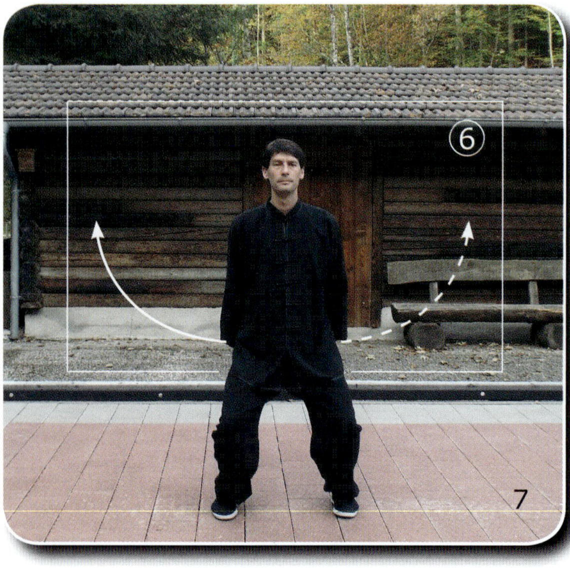

7

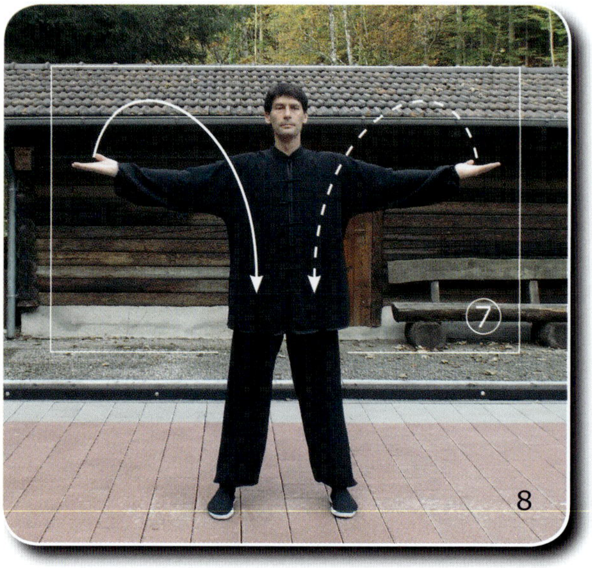

8

4. Die Arme in den Ellbogen beugen und die Hände (Handinnenflächen schauen nach unten, Fingerspitzen zueinander) vor die Brust bringen. Anschließend die Hände vor der Brust nach unten führen. Gleichzeitig dabei die Stellung des Pferdes (MaBu) einnehmen. Siehe Bild 5.
5. — 8. Die gleichen Bewegungen 1 — 4 werden wiederholt. Siehe Bilder 6 - 9. Die Position 4 ist die Ausgangsstellung für die Position 5 (d.h. die Bewegung startet aus dem MaBu).

Die Bewegungen 1 — 8 ein zweites Mal wiederholen. Am Ende des zweiten Durchgangs nur die Hände nach unten führen (d.h. man bleibt aufrecht stehen). Siehe Bild 10. Die Vorstellungskraft wird auf den Punkt YongQuan gerichtet (YiShou YongQuan).

4. Bend your arms at the elbows and guide your hands in front of your chest (your palms pointing downwards, your fingertips towards each other). Then guide your hands down in front of your chest. At the same time take the Position of the Horse (MaBu). See illustration 5.
5.— 8. Repeat the same movements as 1 — 4. See illustrations 6 - 9. Position 4 is the initial position for position 5 (i.e. the movement starts from MaBu).

Repeat the movements 1 — 8 a second time. At the end of the second sequence guide your hands down only (i.e. you keep standing straight). See illustration 10. Your imagination is directed at YongQuan Point (YiShou YongQuan).

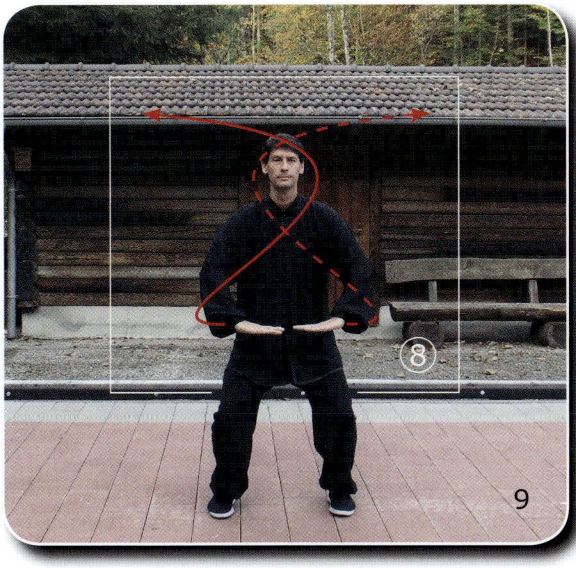


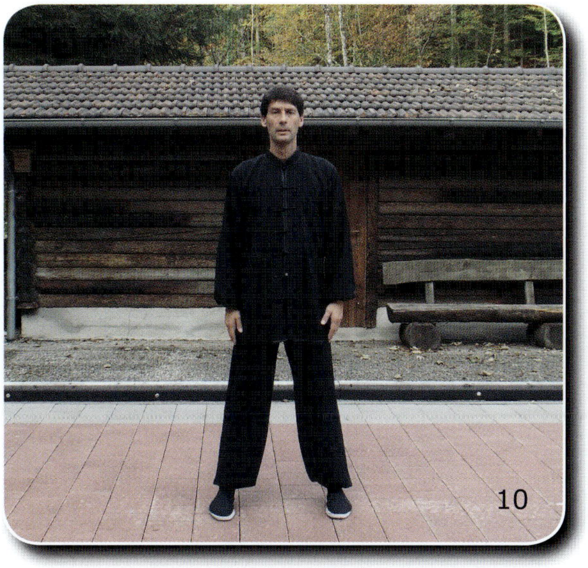

## 七、寿星练武

1、左弓步搂膝冲拳，拳心向下，左右足保持20公分横向距离。（图1，2）

2、重心右移，左足提起向后倒插步，成歇步下蹲，右拳收于腰间，同时左拳变掌由左向上向下压于右胸前（掌心向下）。（图3）

3、身体起立，同时向左后转180度，双拳收于腰间。（图4）

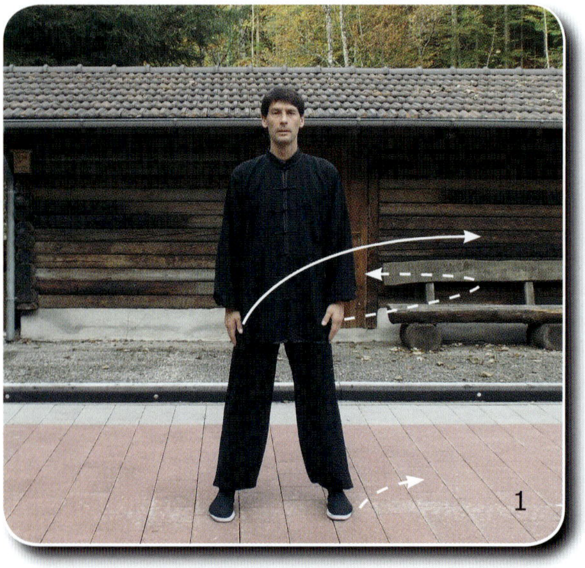


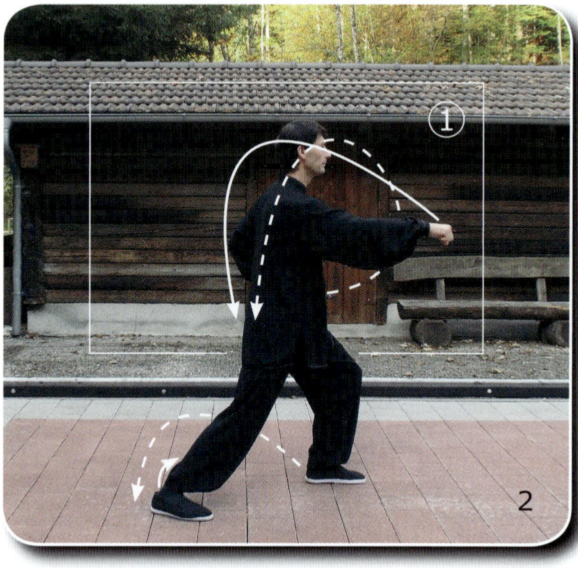


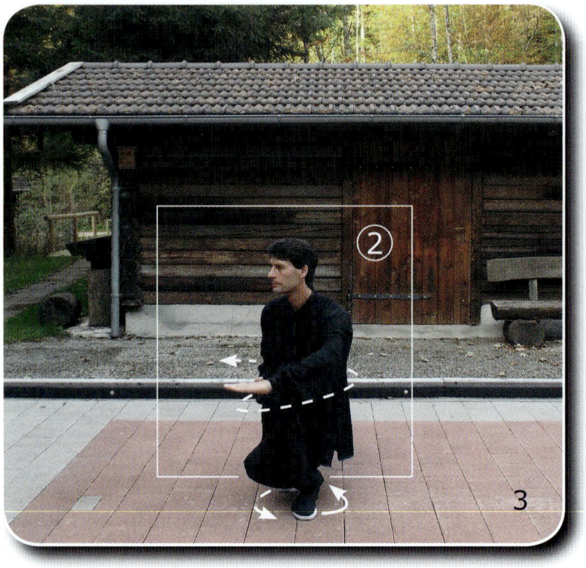


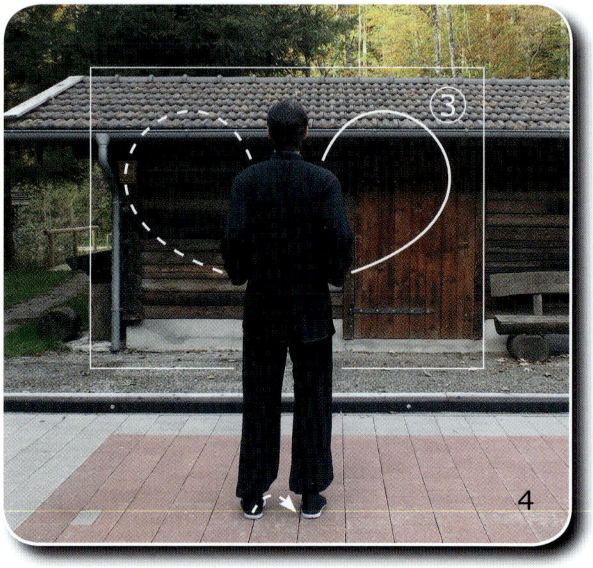

## VII. Der Gott der Langlebigkeit praktiziert die Kampfkunst

1. Den linken Fuß nach links zu einem linken Bogenschritt (GongBu) setzen. Die Breite des GongBu zwischen dem linken und rechten Fuß soll etwa 20 cm betragen. Gleichzeitig mit der linken Hand am Knie vorbeistreifen und sie dann anschließend zur Faust schließen und zur Taille zurückziehen. Während man die linke Faust zur Taille zurückzieht, mit der rechten Faust nach vorne stoßen. Siehe Bilder 1 und 2.
2. Den rechten Fuß auf dem Fußballen nach links drehen (bis der Fuß wieder gerade nach vorne schaut). Dann den Schwerpunkt auf die rechte Seite verlagern. Anschließend den linken Fuß hinter den rechten Fuß setzen und nach unten gehen zur Stellung des Ruhenden Schrittes (XieBu). Dabei die rechte Faust nach oben führen, umdrehen (Handrücken schaut nach unten) und zurück zur rechten Seite der Taille nehmen. Gleichzeitig die linke Faust öffnen und in einem Bogen zuerst nach oben und dann auf der rechten Seite der Brust nach unten drücken. Die Handfläche schaut nach unten. Siehe Bild 3.
3. Den Körper wieder aufrichten und gleichzeitig dabei um 180° nach links drehen. Dabei die linke Hand zur Faust schließen und zur Taille zurückziehen. Beide Fäuste befinden sich nun seitlich an der Taille (die Faustrücken schauen nach unten). Siehe Bild 4.

## VII. The God of Longevity Practises Martial Art

1. Put your left foot to the left hand side to a Bow Step (GongBu) at the left hand side. The breadth of GongBu between your left and right foot should measure 20 cm. At the same time brush along your knee with your left hand and afterwards close it into a fist and guide it back to your waist. While drawing your left fist back to your waist punch forwards with your right fist. See illustrations 1 and 2.
2. Turn your right foot to the left on the ball of your foot (until your foot points straight forward again). Then shift your centre of gravity to the right hand side. Following this put your left foot behind your right foot and go down to the Position of Resting Step (XieBu). In doing so guide your right fist upwards, turn it (the back of your hand pointing downwards) and take it back to the right hand side of your waist. At the same time open your left fist and in a bow push it first upwards and then downwards at the right hand side of your chest. Your palm points downwards. See illustration 3.
3. Straighten your body again and at the same time turn it by 180° to the left. In doing so close your left hand into a fist and draw it back towards your waist. Both your fists are now situated at the sides of your waist (the backs of your fists pointing downwards). See illustration 4.

4、双拳变掌，经侧平举胸前下按，左足向右足靠拢。（图5）
5—8动同1—4动，其方向相反。（图6—9）

第二个8拍，同第一个8拍。意守丹田。

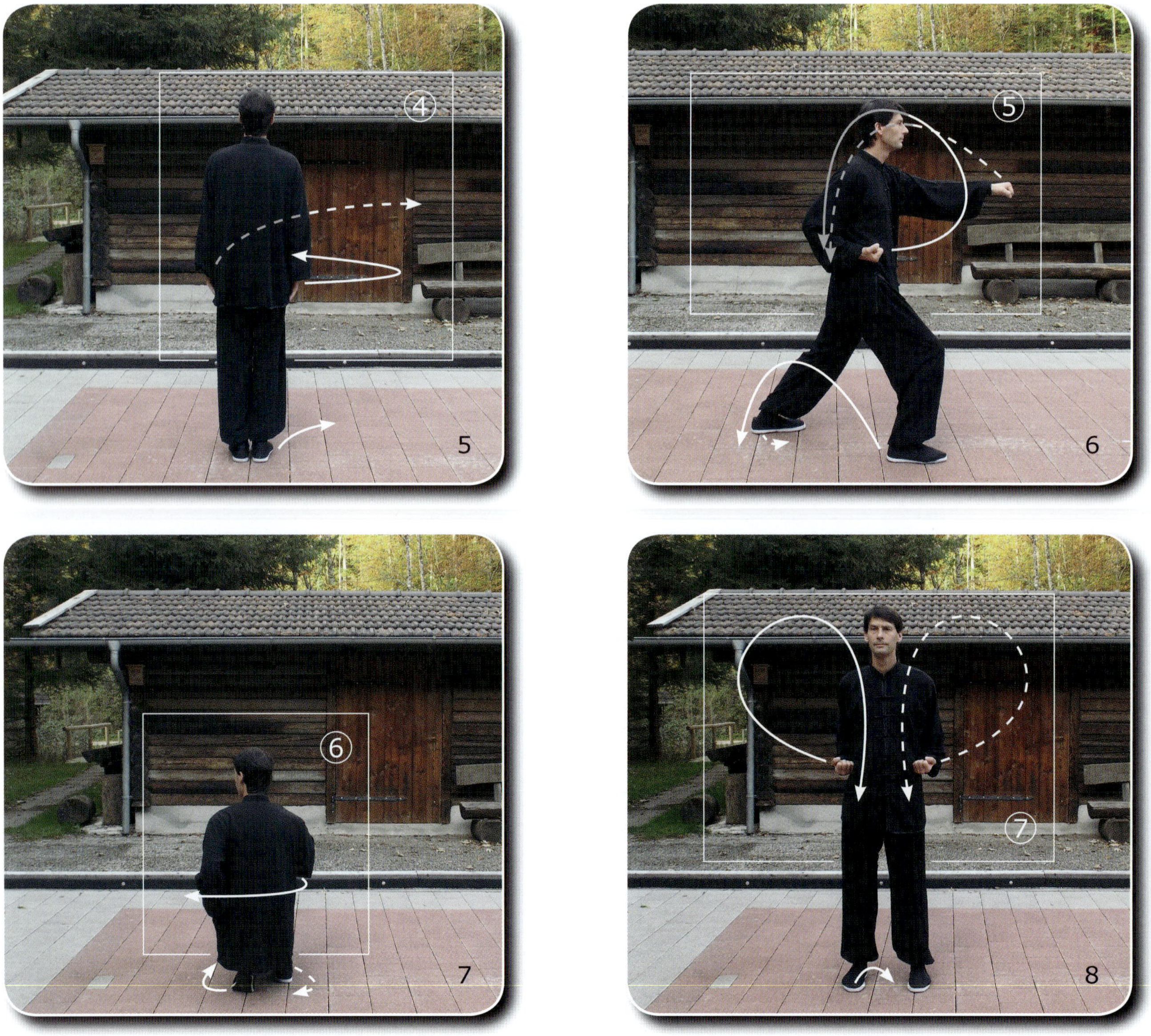

4. Die Fäuste öffnen und die Hände bogenförmig zu den Seiten und nach oben bringen. Anschließend die Hände (Handflächen schauen nach unten) vor der Brust nach unten drücken. Gleichzeitig dabei den linken Fuß zum rechten Fuß heransetzen. Siehe Bild 5.
5. — 8. Die gleichen Bewegungen 1 — 4 zur anderen Seite ausführen. Siehe Bilder 6 - 9.

Die Bewegungen 1 — 8 ein zweites Mal wiederholen. Die Vorstellungskraft wird auf das DanTian gerichtet (YiShou DanTian).

4. Open your fists and guide your hands to your sides and upwards in a bow. Then push your hands downwards in front of your chest (your palms pointing downwards). At the same time put your left foot next to your right foot. See illustration 5.
5. — 8. Carry out the same movements 1 — 4 to the other side. See illustrations 6 - 9.

Repeat the movements a second time. Your imagination is directed at DanTian (YiShou DanTian).

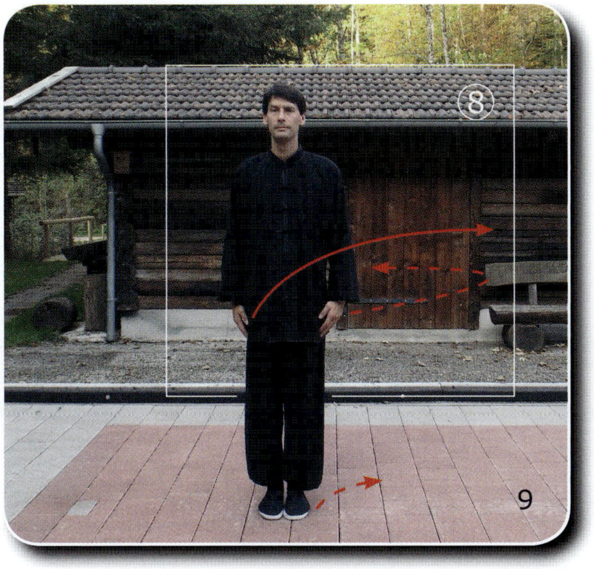

## 八、孔雀开屏

1、双手变勾手，向体侧上摆至水平，同时双足跟提起。（图1, 2）
2、两手变掌下按，手心向下，同时两腿下蹲。（图3）
3、双手变掌直臂交叉上举，边抖动手腕边向两侧打开，同时左足后摆，足尖点地。（图4）

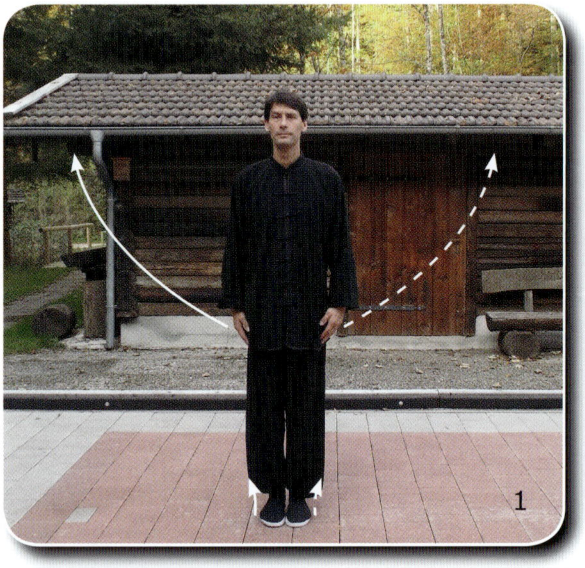


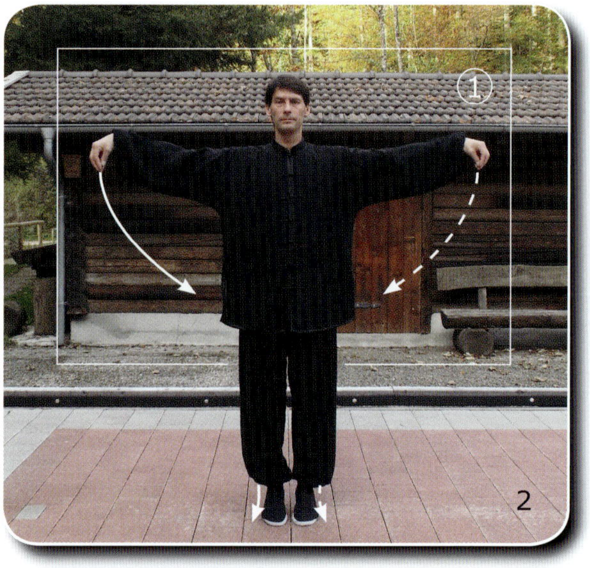


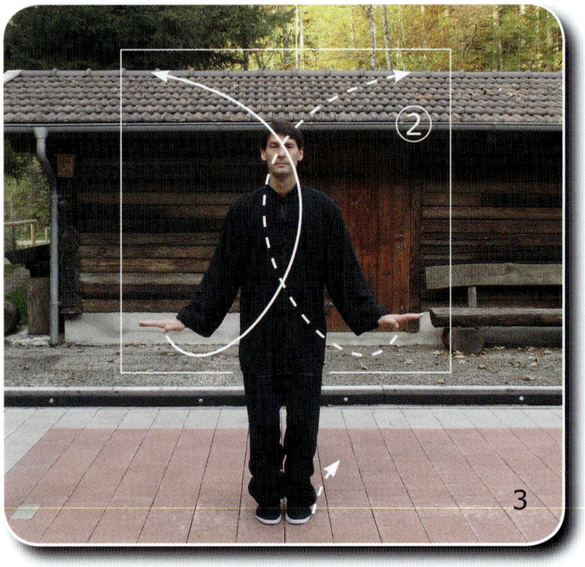


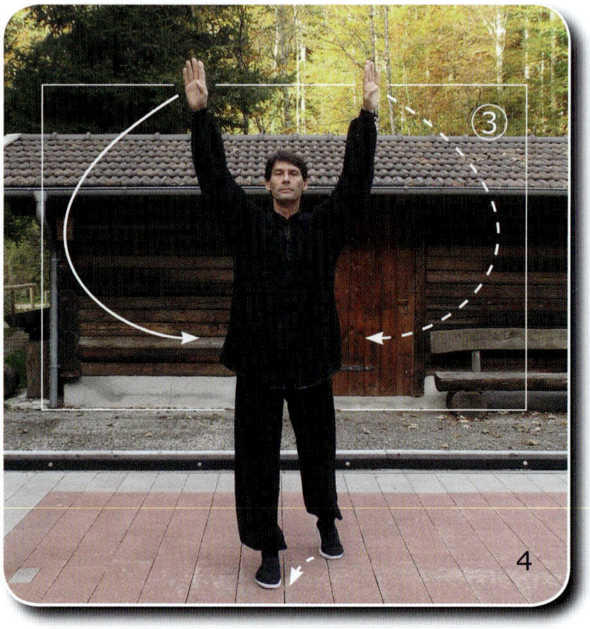

## VIII. Der Pfau öffnet seine Flügel und schlägt das Rad

1. Die Finger und Daumen zur Hakenhand (GouShou) schließen (d. h. die Spitzen des Daumens und der Finger werden zusammengebracht und das Handgelenk nach unten gebeugt) und an den Seiten nach oben bringen in die Waagerechte. Gleichzeitig dabei die Fersen anheben. Siehe Bilder 1 und 2.
2. Die Hände öffnen und nach unten drücken zur linken und rechten Körperseite. Die Handflächen zeigen dabei nach unten. Gleichzeitig die Knie beugen. Siehe Bild 3.
3. Die Arme zur Mitte führen, überkreuzen und weiter nach oben und wieder auseinander führen. Dabei zeigen die Handgelenke nach außen und die Hände vibrieren. Gleichzeitig den linken Fuß nach hinten strecken. Die linke Fußspitze berührt dabei den Boden. Siehe Bild 4.

## VIII. The Peacock Opens Its Wings and Spreads Its Tail

1. Shut your fingers and your thumbs to Hookhand (GouShou), putting the tips of your thumbs and fingers together and bending down your wrists and guide them up at your sides to the horizontal line. At the same time lift your heels. See illustrations 1 and 2.
2. Open your hands and push them downwards towards the left and right hand sides of your body. Your palms point downwards. At the same time bend your knees. See illustration 3.
3. Guide your arms to the middle, cross them and guide them further up and apart again. In doing so your wrists point sideways and your hands vibrate. At the same time stretch your left foot backwards. Your left tiptoe touches the ground in doing so. See illustration 4.

4、左足收回，两腿下蹲。（与2动相同）（图5）
5—8动同1—4动。（3与7动交换腿后摆起点地）（图6—9）

第二个8拍，同第一个8拍，后摆腿可以腾空，足尖不点地。（图10）共做两个8拍。最后一拍成预备式。（图11）意守命门。

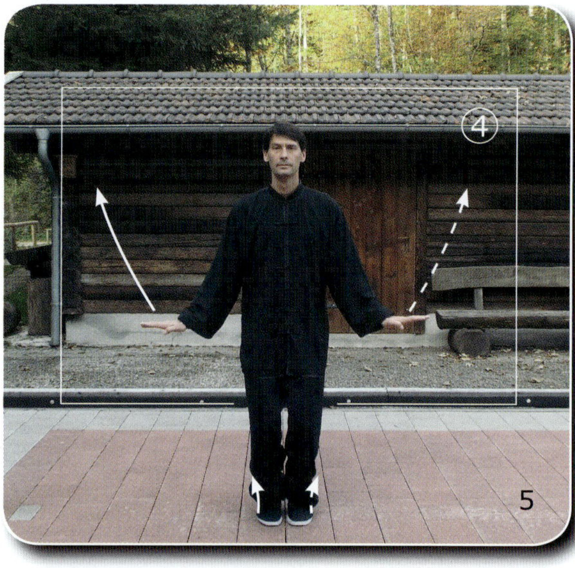

5

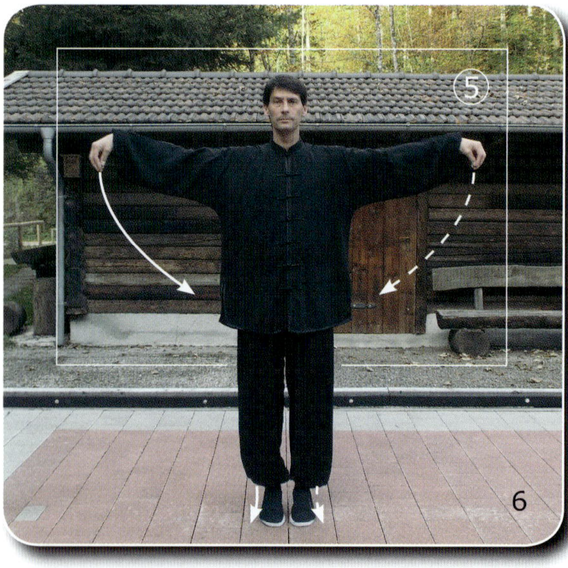

6

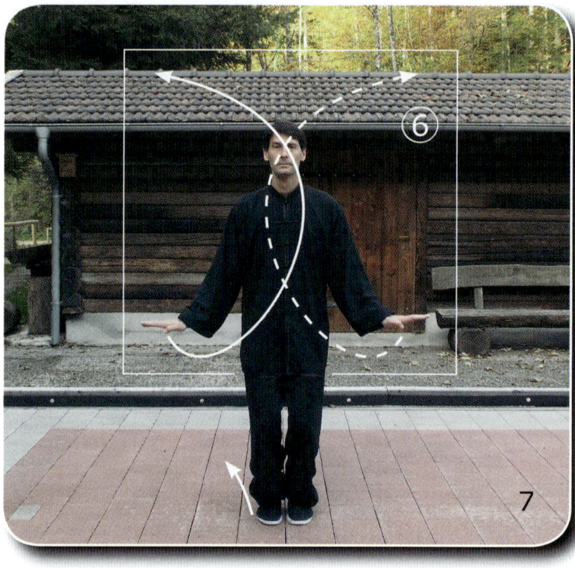

7

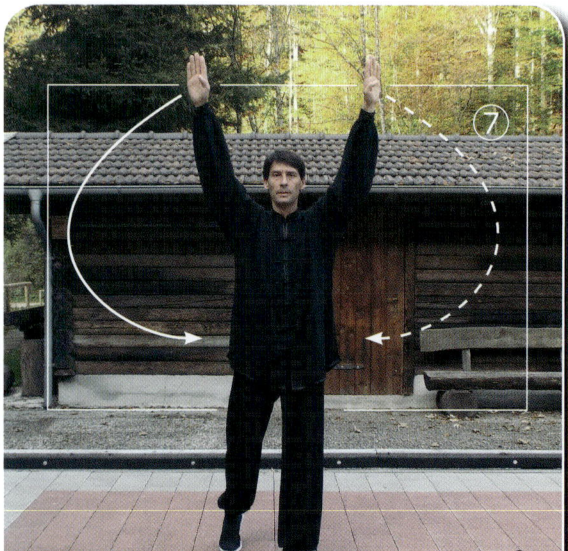

8

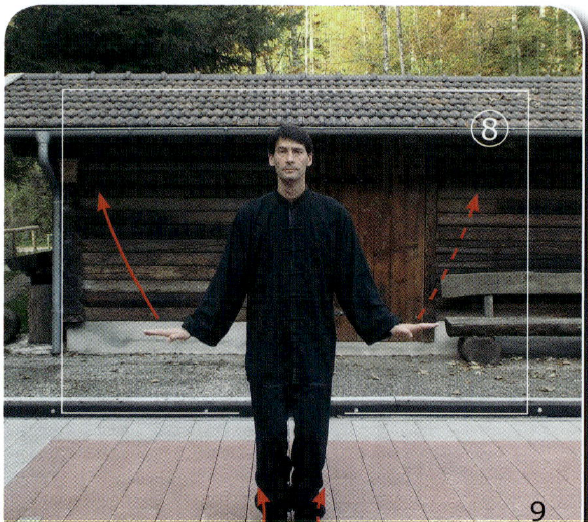

9

4. Den linken Fuß wieder an den rechten Fuß heransetzen und anschließend die Knie beugen. Beim Beugen der Knie die Arme nach unten drücken (wie Bewegung 2). Siehe Bild 5.
5. — 8. Die gleichen Bewegungen 1 — 4 wiederholen. Nur bei Punkt 7 den rechten Fuß nach hinten strecken (statt den linken Fuß wie bei Punkt 3). Siehe Bilder 6 - 9.

Die Bewegungen 1 — 8 ein zweites Mal wiederholen. Bei den Punkten 3 und 7 kann der Fuß auch angehoben werden. Siehe Bild 10. Bei der letzten Bewegung nicht die Knie beugen, nur die Arme in die Ausgangsposition zurückbringen. Siehe Bild 11. Die Vorstellungskraft wird auf den Punkt MingMen gerichtet (YiShou MingMen).

4. Guide your left foot back to your right foot and then bend your knees. When bending your knees push your arms downwards (like movement 2). See illustration 5.
5. — 8. Repeat the same movements 1 — 4. Only in point 7 stretch your right foot back (instead of your left foot as in point 3). See illustrations 6 - 9.

Repeat the movements 1 — 8 a second time. At points 3 and 7 your foot may also be lifted. See illustration 10. During the last movement do not bend your knees, but only take your arms back into the initial position. See illustration 11. Your imagination is directed at MingMen Point (YiShou MingMen).

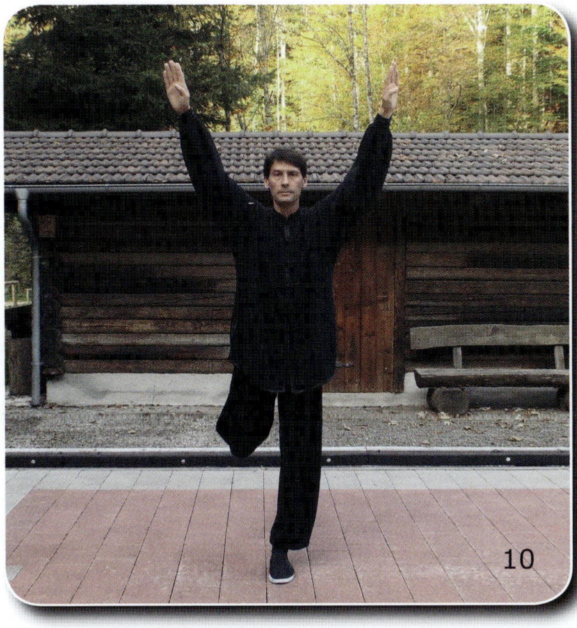
10

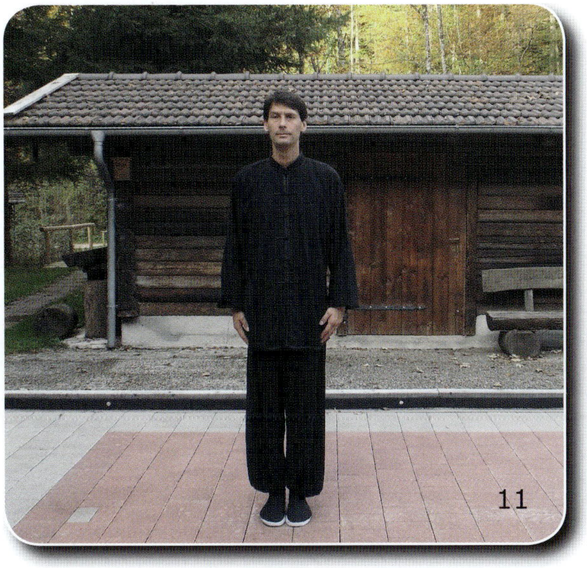
11

## 九、踏步展掌

第一个8拍:

踏步摆臂（左足开始），每逢左足踏步为一拍，共做4拍。（图1—3）

从第5拍开始，双足踏步不变，两手摆动改为内旋翻腕，向两侧外拔展手掌。共做4拍。（图4—6）

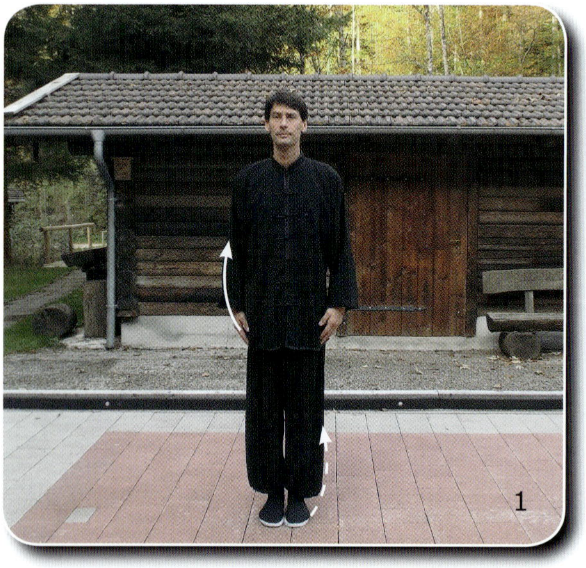


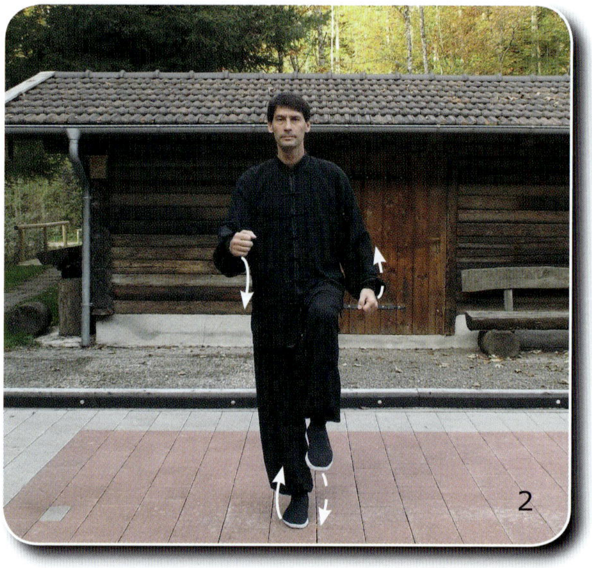


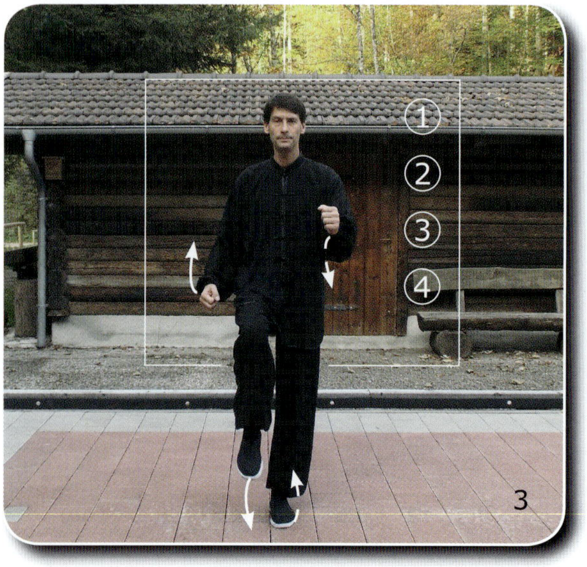


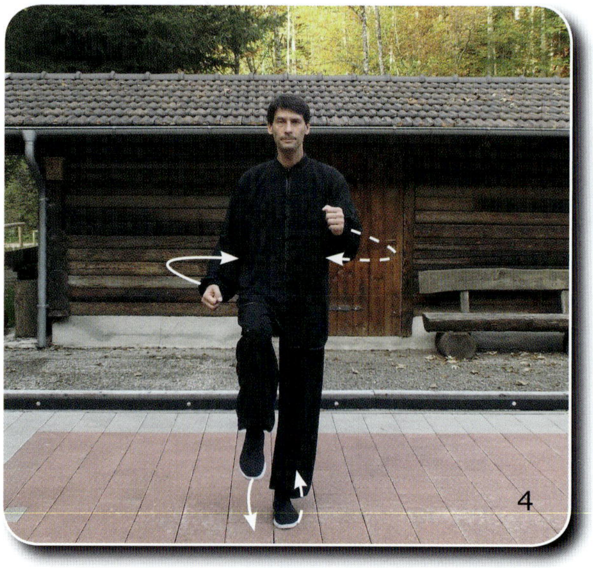

## IX. Auf der Stelle treten und die Hände öffnen

1. — 4. Am Platz zuerst den linken Fuß heben und den rechten Arm nach vorne oben bewegen, dann den rechten Fuß und den linken Arm. Das ist ein Takt. Insgesamt vier solche Takte ausführen. Die Hände sind dabei zu einer lockeren Faust geschlossen. Siehe Bilder 1 - 3.
5. — 8. Die Beinbewegungen bleiben gleich wie bei 1 — 4. Die Hände öffnen und nach innen oben drehen (Handflächen schauen nach oben). Anschließend die Hände zur linken und rechten Seite des Körpers schwingen. Das ist ein Takt. Insgesamt vier solche Takte ausführen. Siehe Bilder 4 - 6.

## IX. Step at the Same Spot and Open Your Hands

1. — 4. Keep standing on the spot and first lift your left foot and move your right arm to the front and up, then your right foot and your left arm. This is one beat. All in all, you carry out four of these beats. Your hands are closed to a light fist while doing so. See illustrations 1 - 3.
5. — 8. The movements of your legs remain the same as in 1 — 4. Open your hands and turn them inwards and upwards (your palms pointing upwards). Next swing your hands to the left and right hand sides of your body. This is one beat. All in all, carry out four such beats. See illustrations 4 - 6.

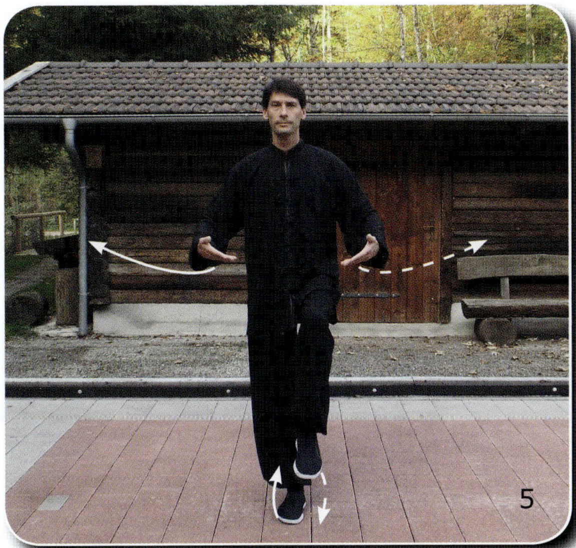


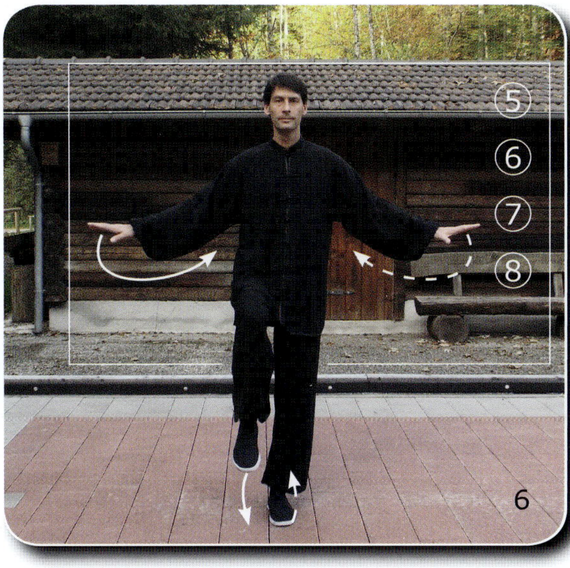

第二个8拍同第一个8拍。

最后做第八拍时，当右足着地时以双手由上而下按掌，并同时大声发出“嗨！”，为练功结束。（图7—12）意守丹田。

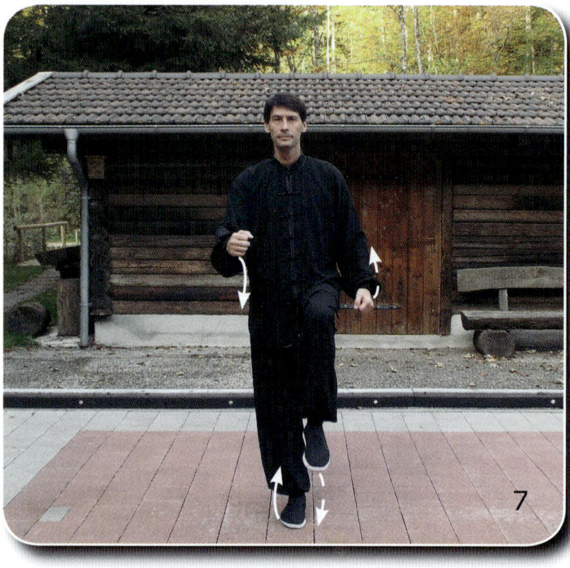


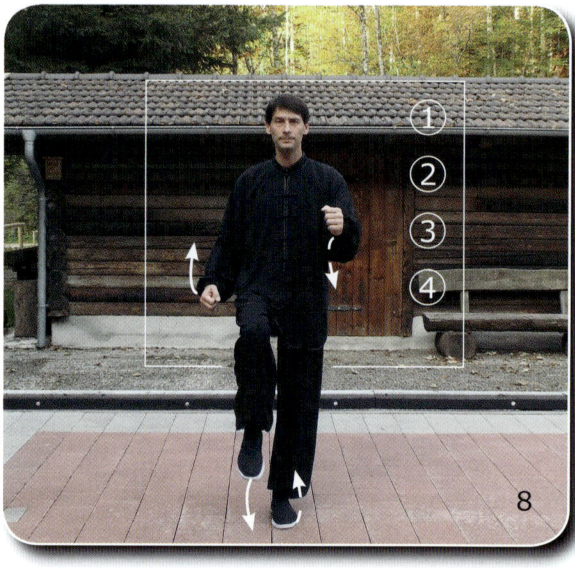


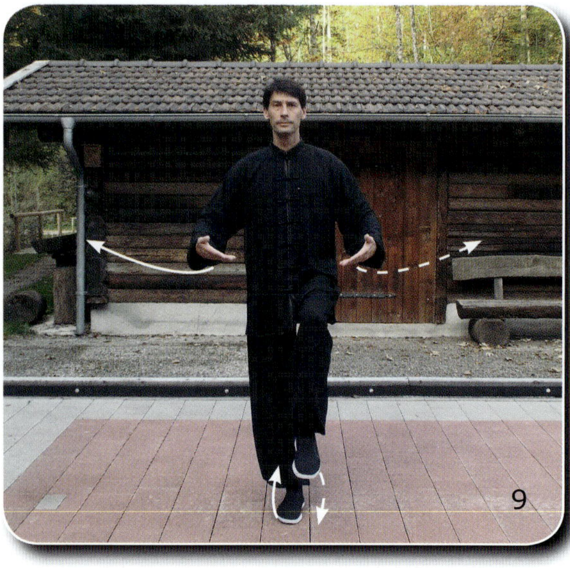


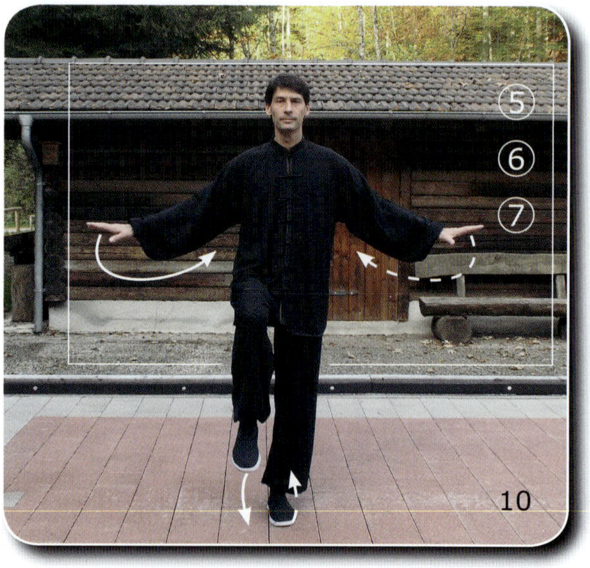

Die Bewegungen 1 — 8 ein zweites Mal wiederholen. Beim letzten Takt des zweiten Durchgangs die Hände nach außen und oben (bis auf Kopfhöhe) führen. Gleichzeitig den rechten Fuß aufsetzen. Dann die Hände vor der Brust nach unten führen, Fingerspitzen einander zugewendet, zur Ausgangsposition. Das nach unten Führen der Hände wird begleitet durch den Laut „Hei", der auch die gesamte Übung des „Sehnen- und Knochen-QiGongs" beendet. Siehe Bilder 7 - 12. Die Vorstellungskraft wird auf das DanTian gerichtet (YiShou DanTian).

Repeat the movements 1 — 8 a second time. During the last beat of the second sequence guide your hands outwards and up (to head height). At the same time put your right foot on the ground. Then guide your hands downwards in front of your chest, the tips of your fingers facing each other, to the initial position. The movement of guiding your hands downwards is accompanied by the sound "Hei" which also puts an end to the complete exercise of the "Sinews and Bones - QiGong". See illustrations 7 - 12. Your imagination is directed at DanTian (YiShou DanTian).

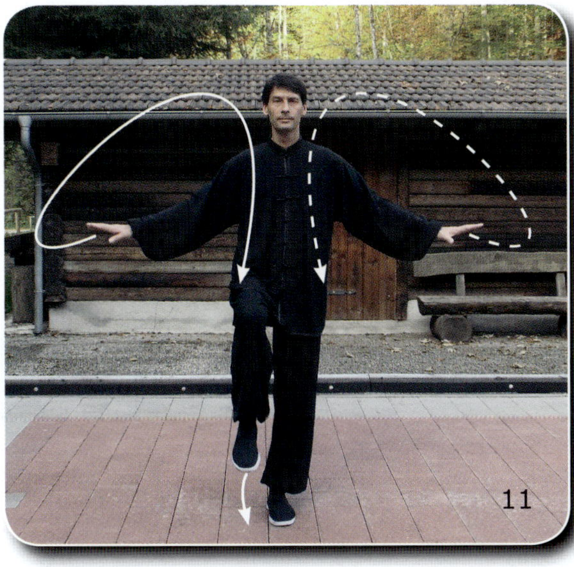
11

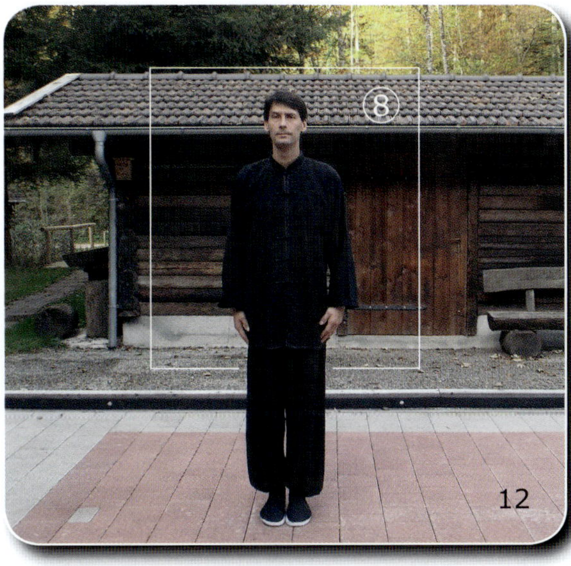

12

## 练习动作全图

## Übersicht der Übungen



## Survey of the Exercises

## 一、太公行书
## I. Der alte Herr übt Kalligraphie
## I. The Old Gentleman Practises Calligraphy

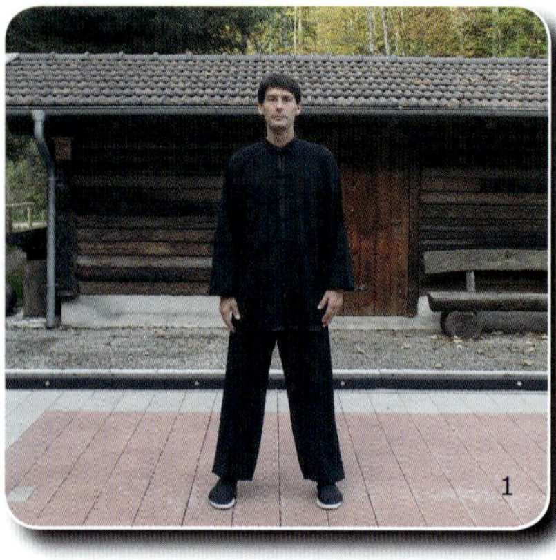
1

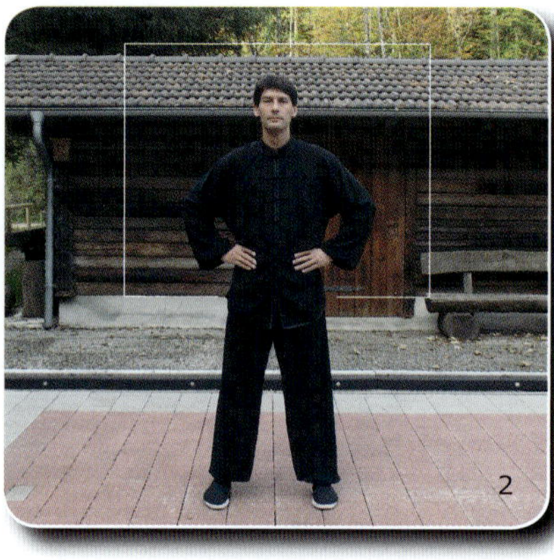
2

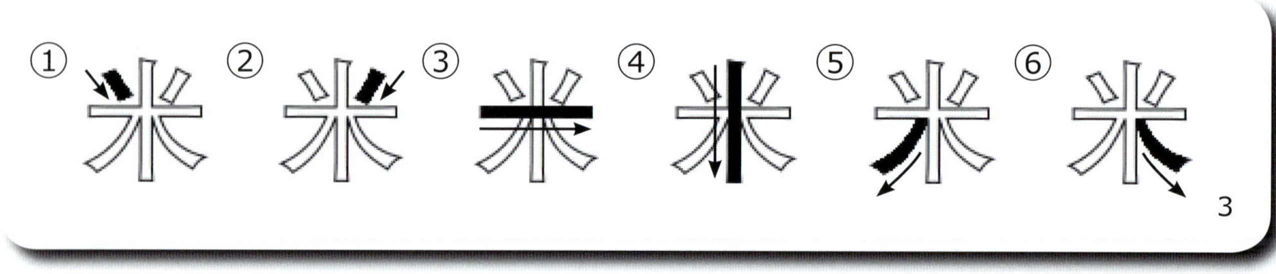

3

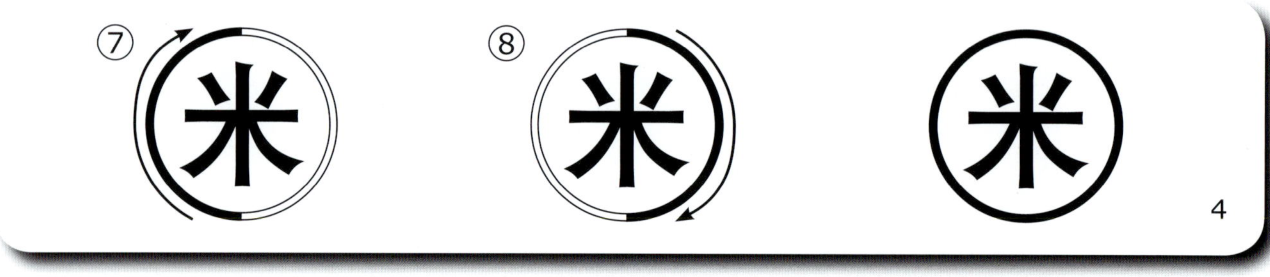

4

## 二、多面推掌

## II. Die Handflächen in mehrere Richtungen schieben

## II. Shove Your Palms into Several Directions

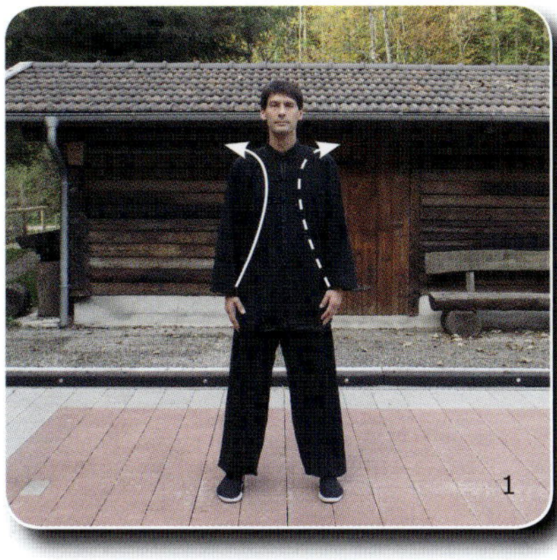


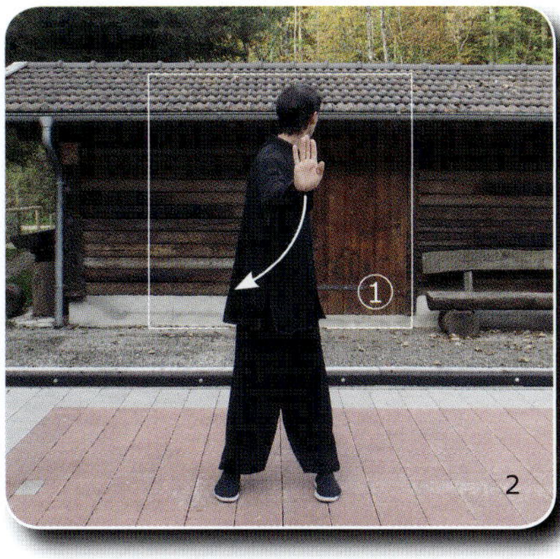


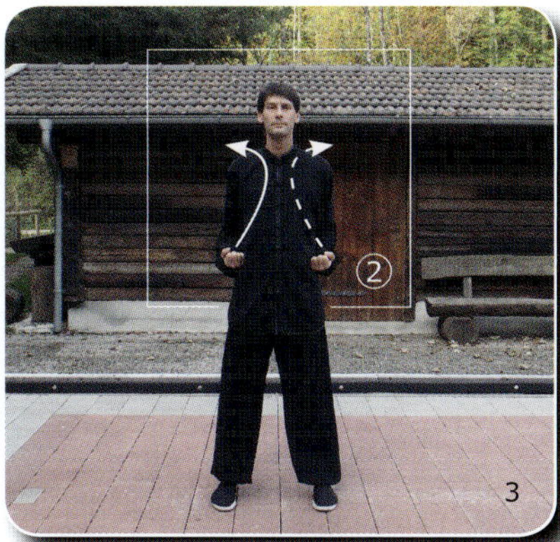


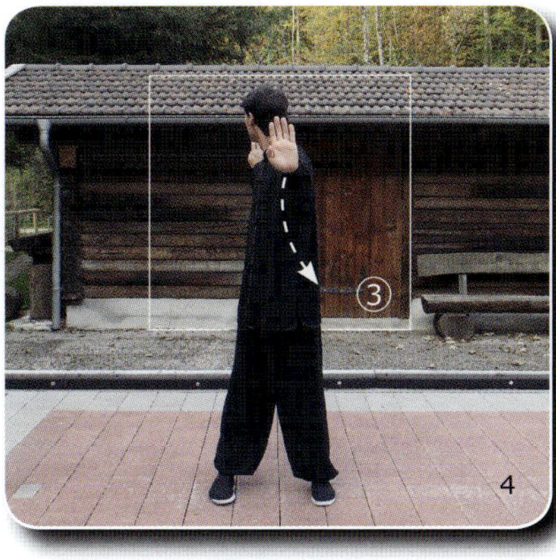


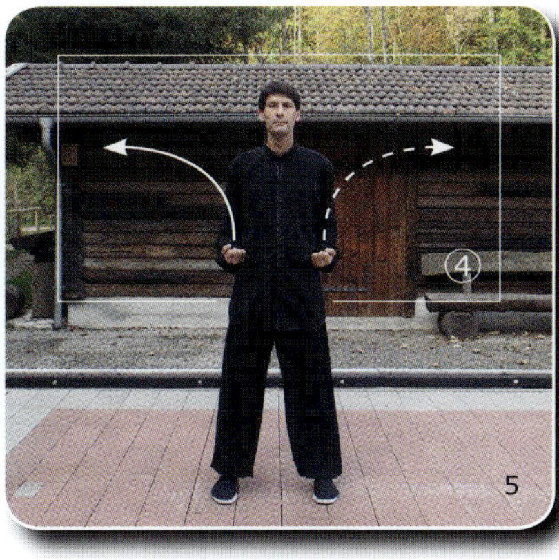


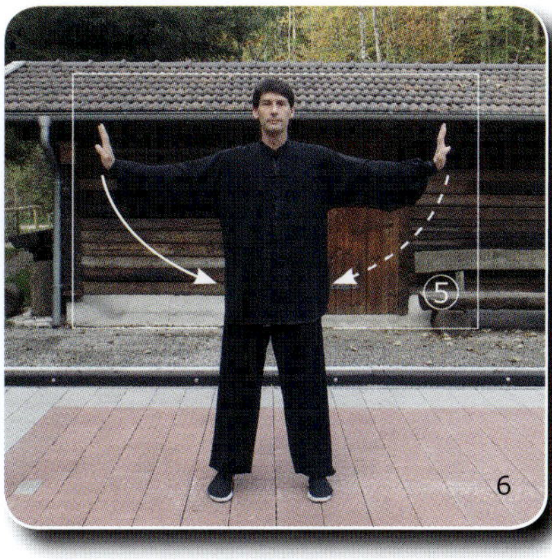


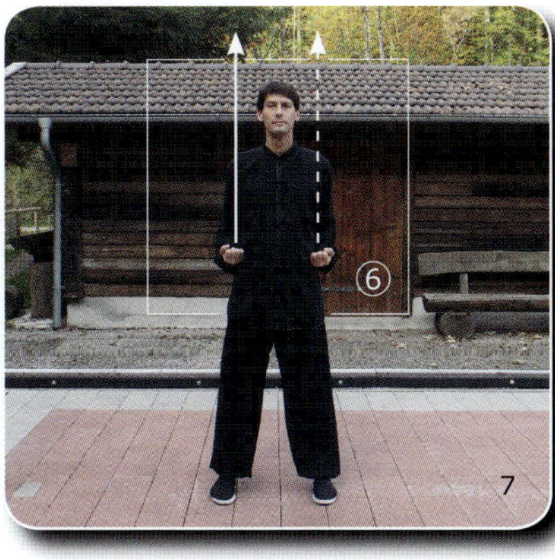


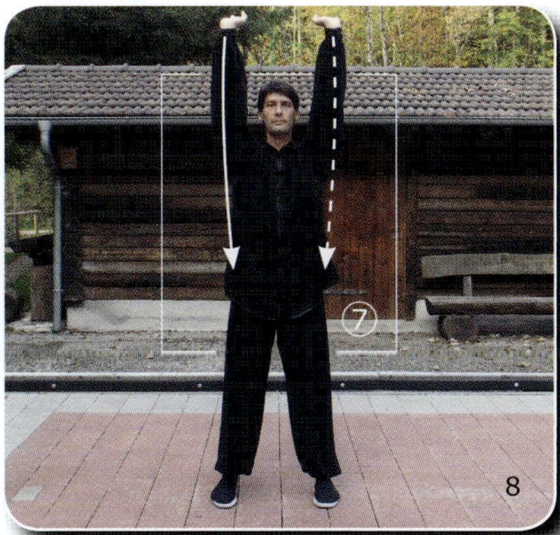


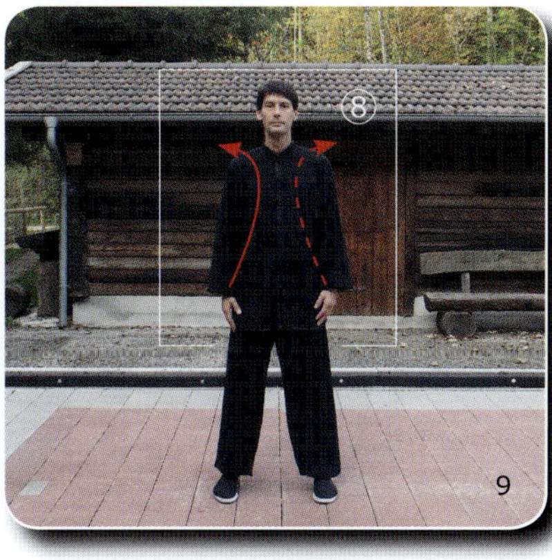

## 三、 握拳下蹲

## III. Fäuste machen und die Knie beugen

## III. Make Fists and Bend Your Knees

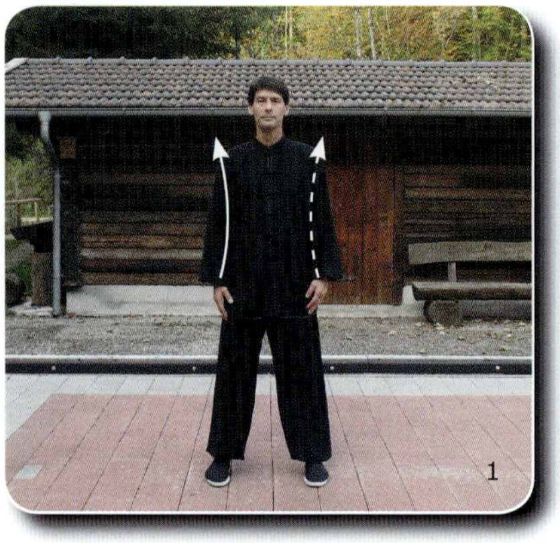


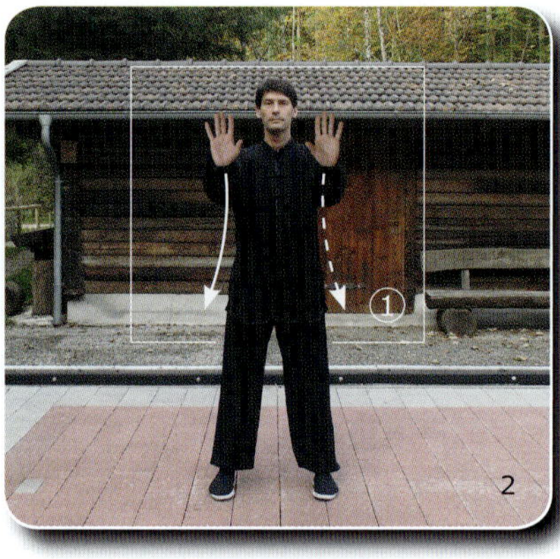


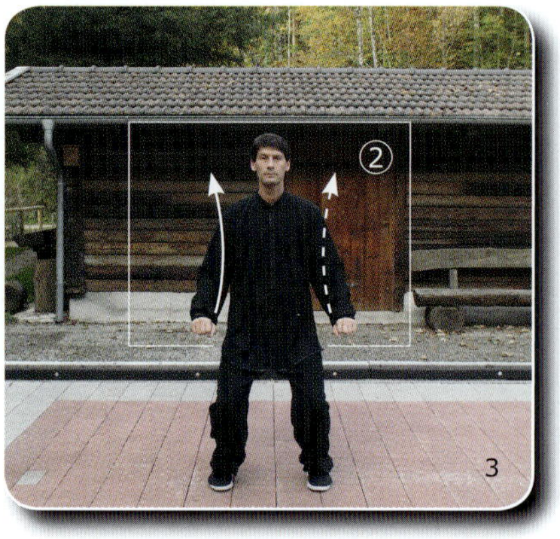


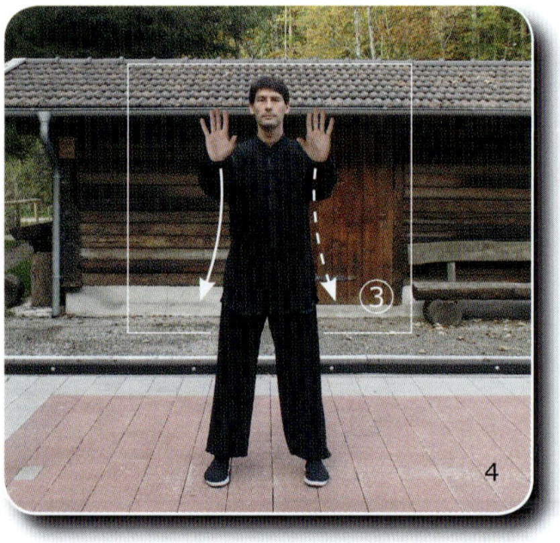


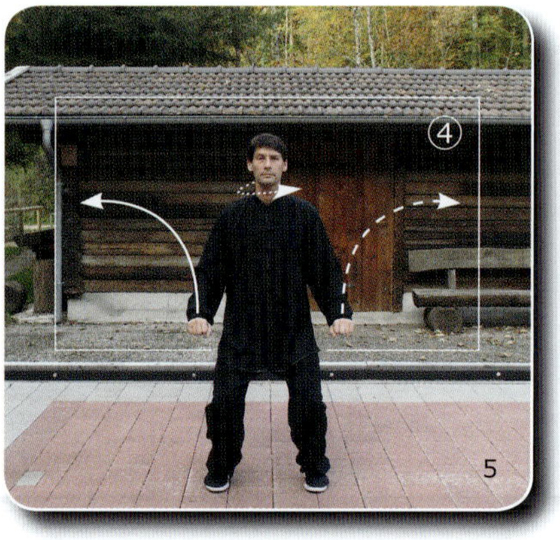


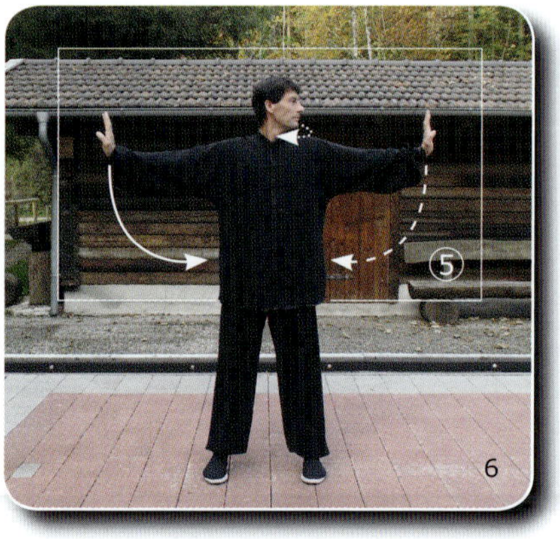


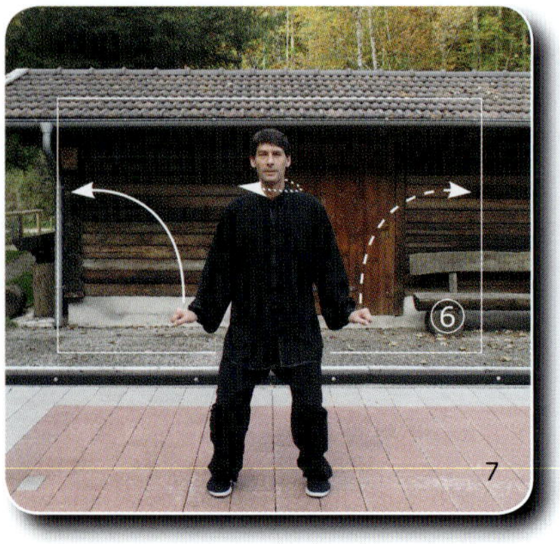


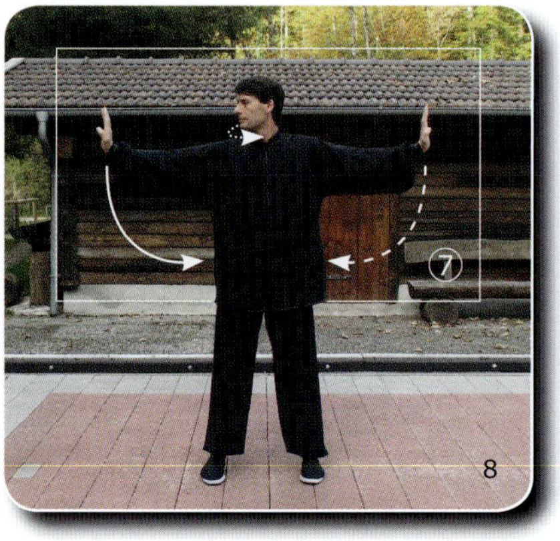


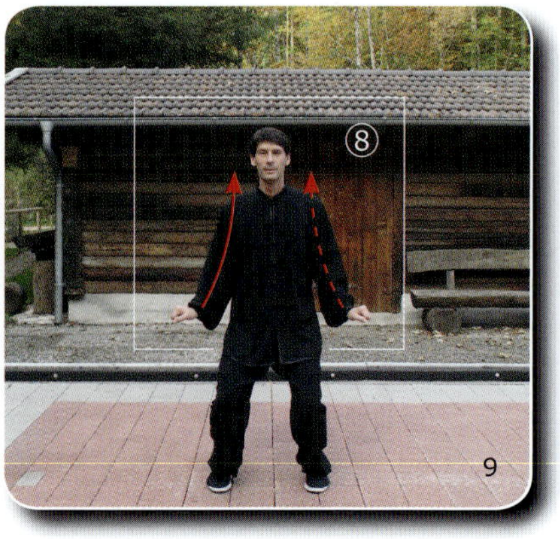

## 四、展臂舒胸

## IV. Die Arme öffnen und die Brust herausstrecken

## IV. Open Your Arms and Spread Your Chest

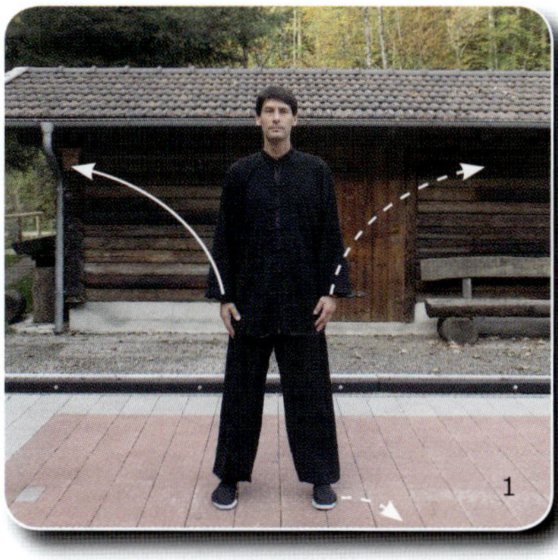


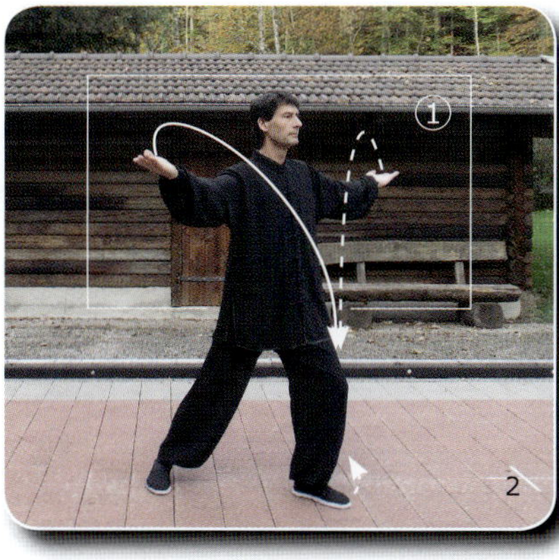


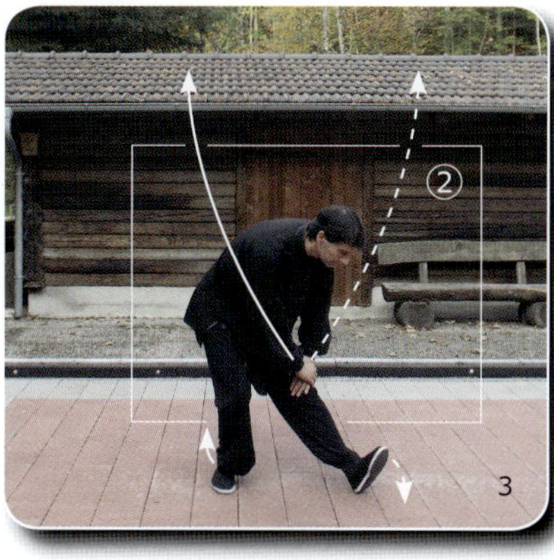


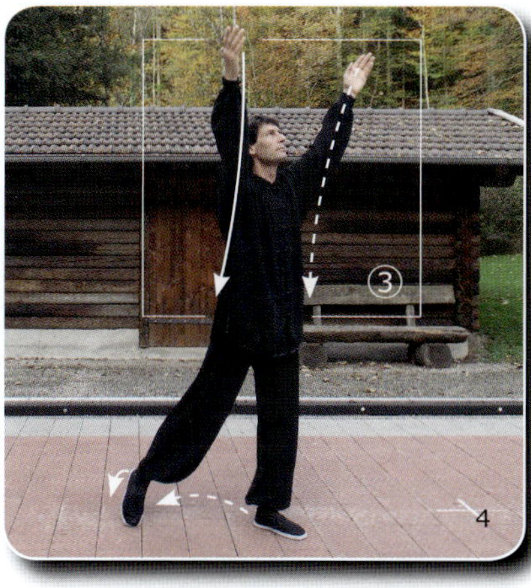


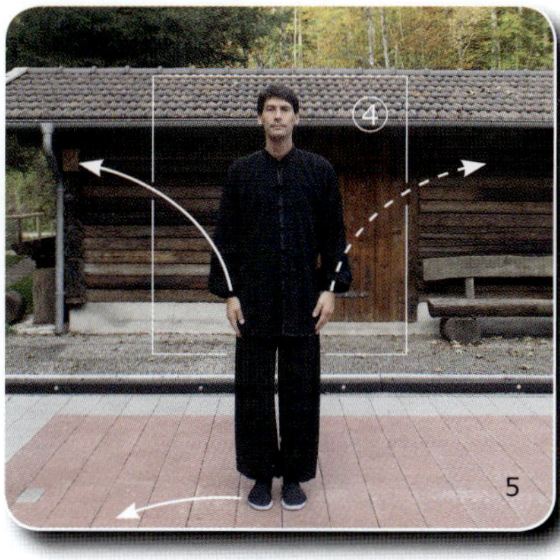


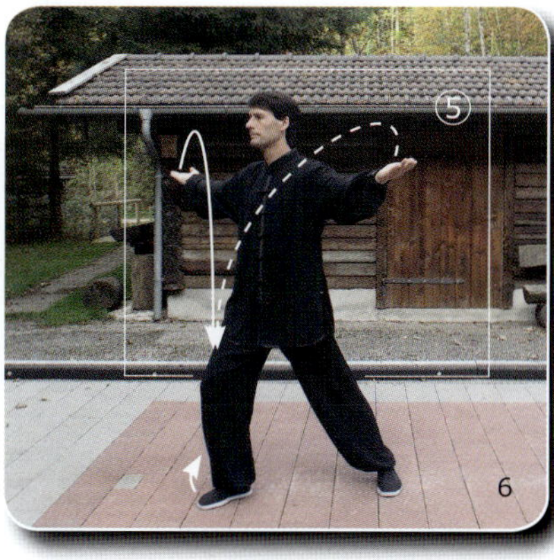


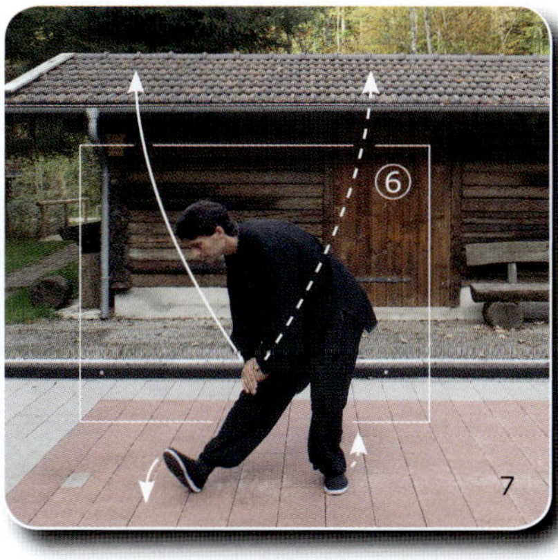


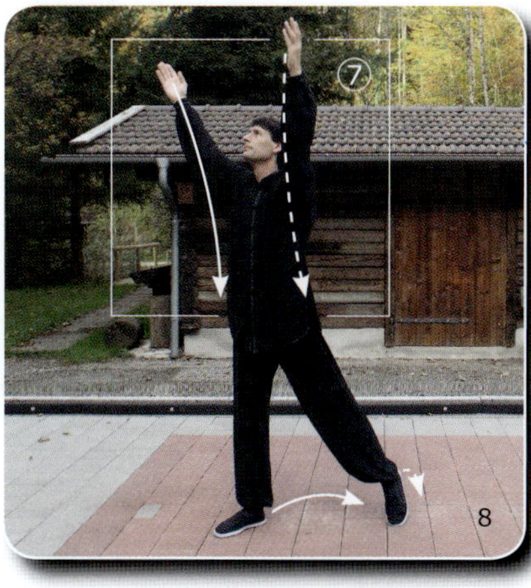


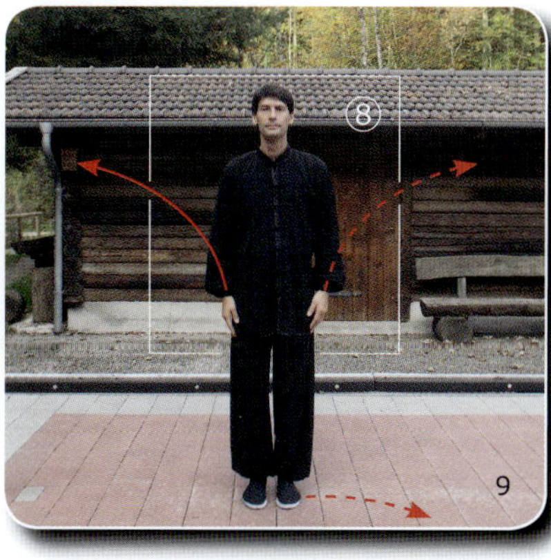

## 五、拙童脱衣

## V. Ein unbeholfenes Kind zieht seine Kleidung aus

## V. A Clumsy Child Takes off Its Garments

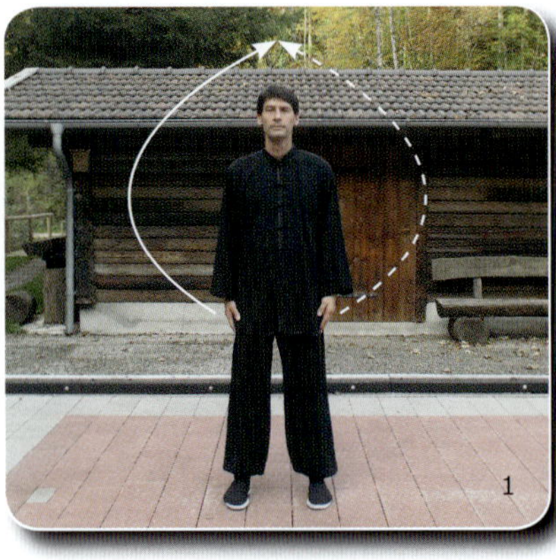


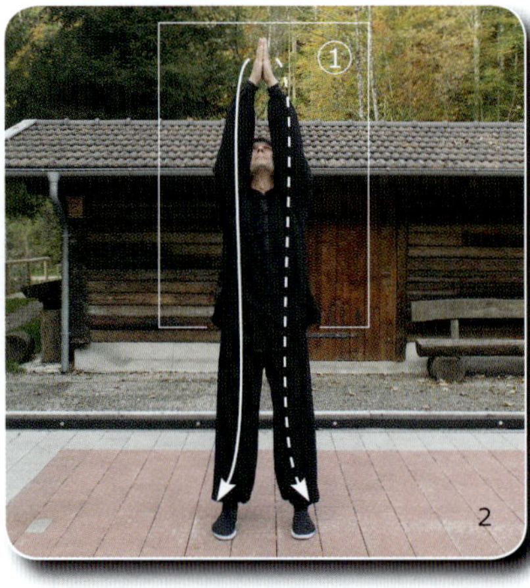


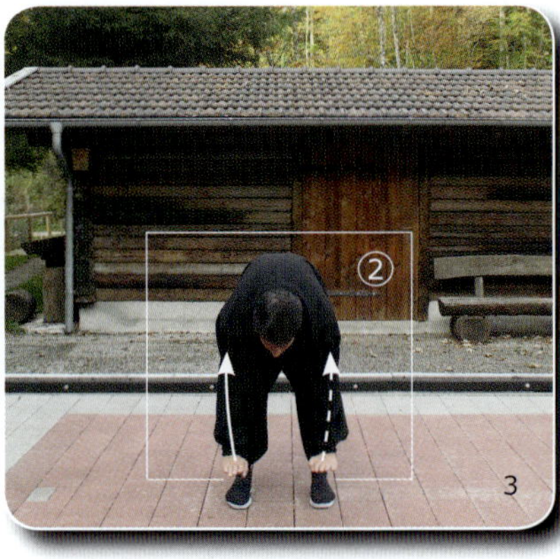


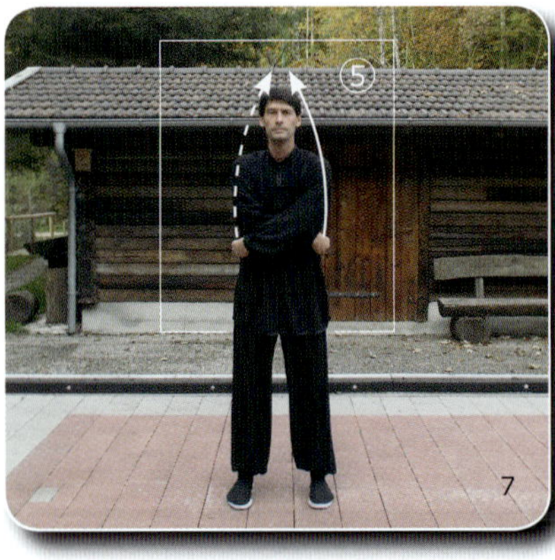


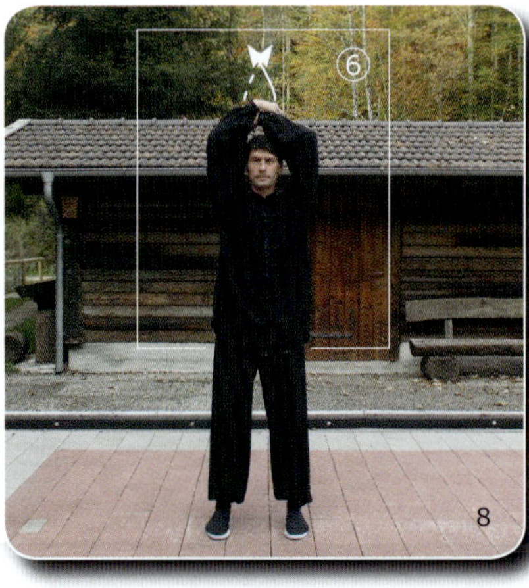


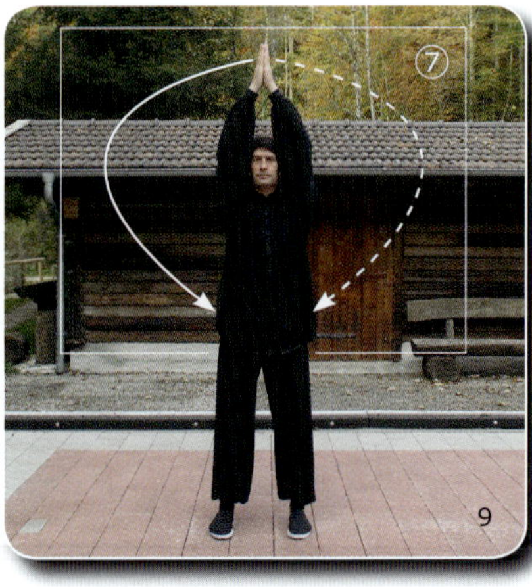

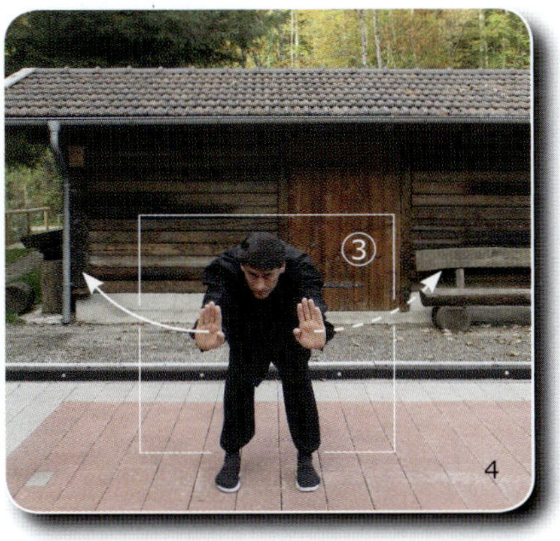
③
4

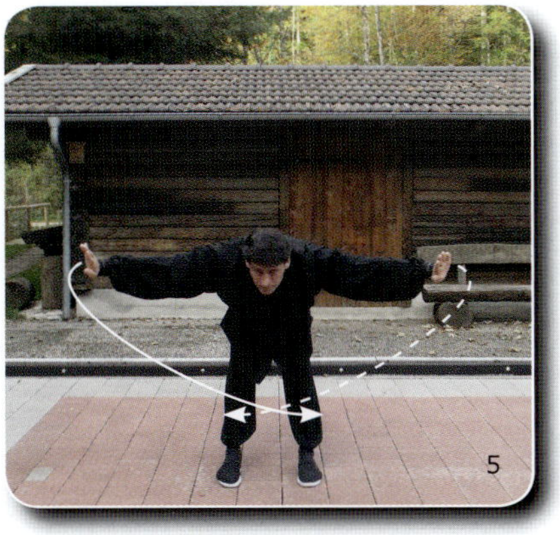
5

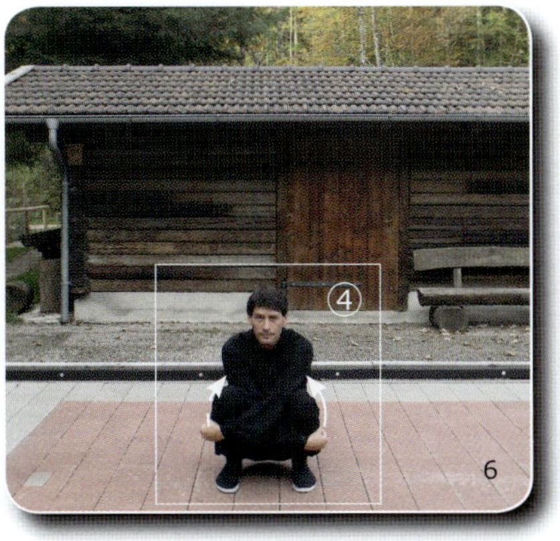
④
6

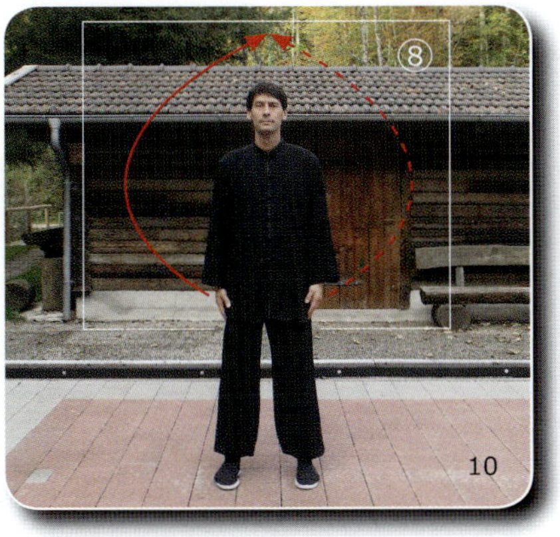
⑧
10

## 六、震撼大地
## VI. Die Erde schütteln
## VI. Shake the Ground

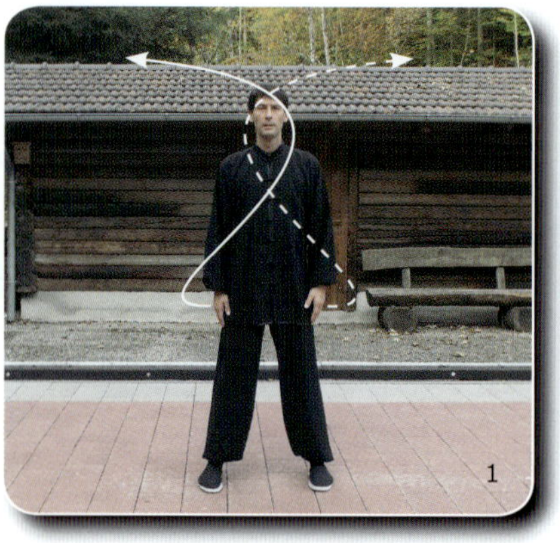


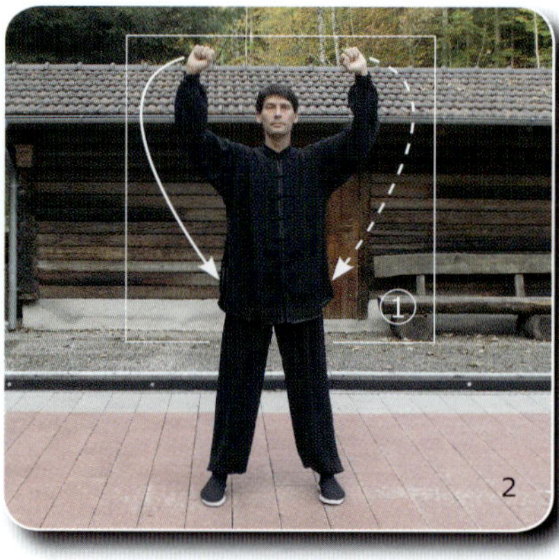


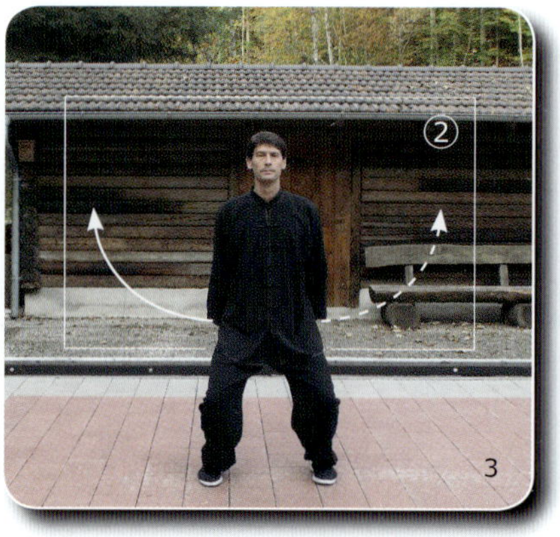


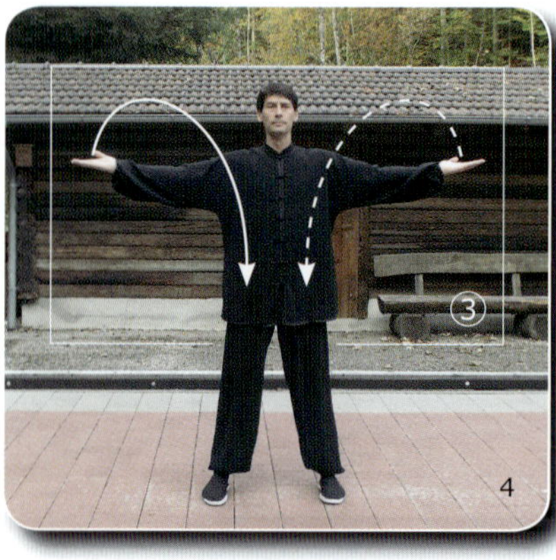


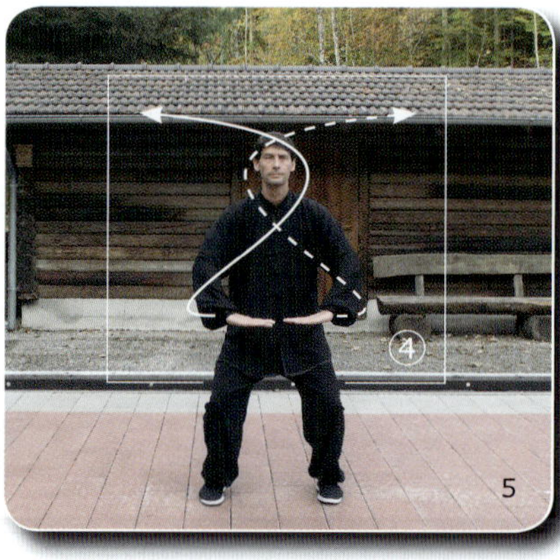


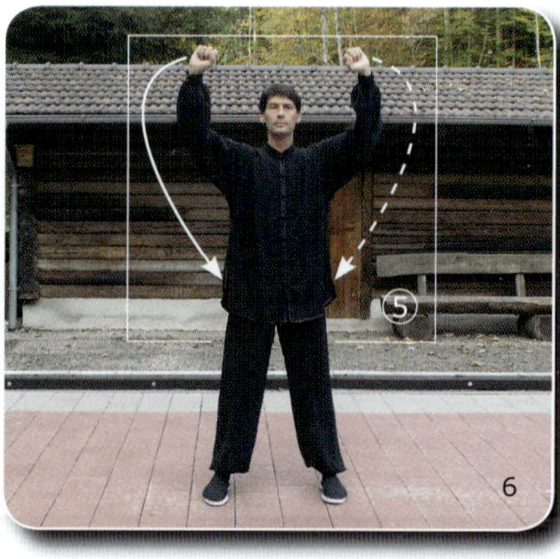


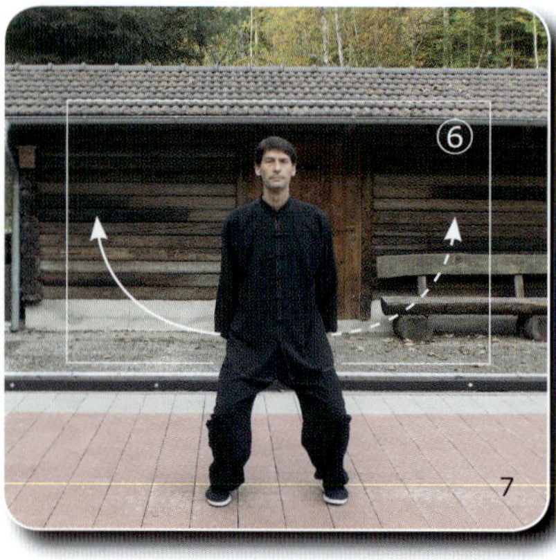


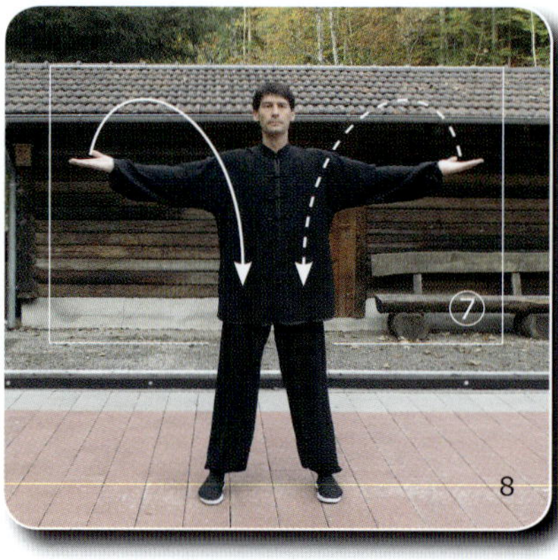


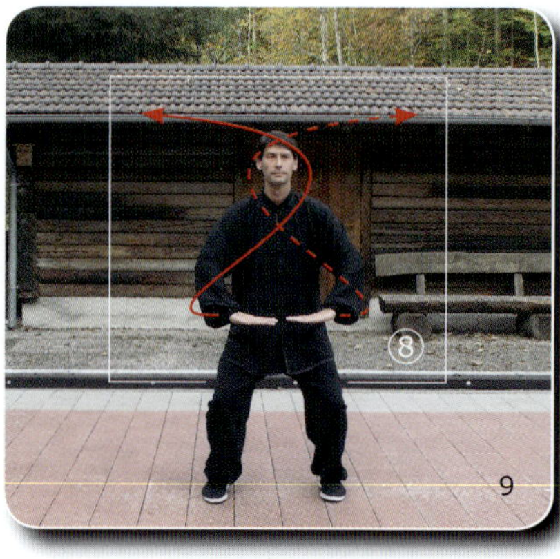

## 七、寿星练武

## VII. Der Gott der Langlebigkeit praktiziert die Kampfkunst

## VII. The God of Longevity Practises Martial Art

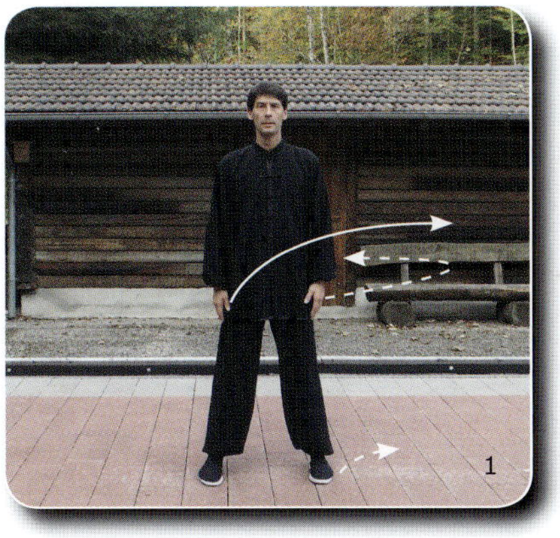


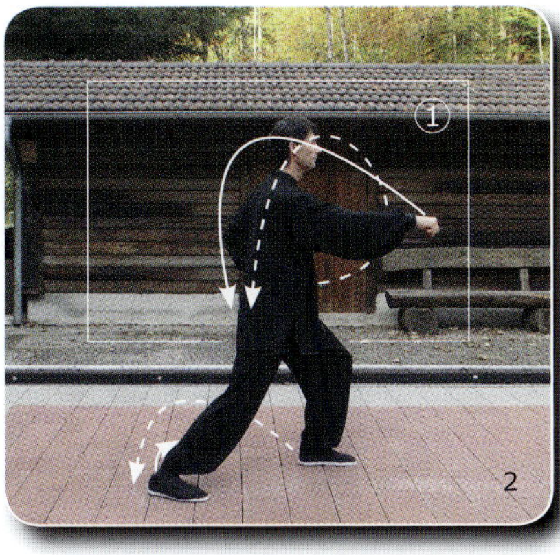


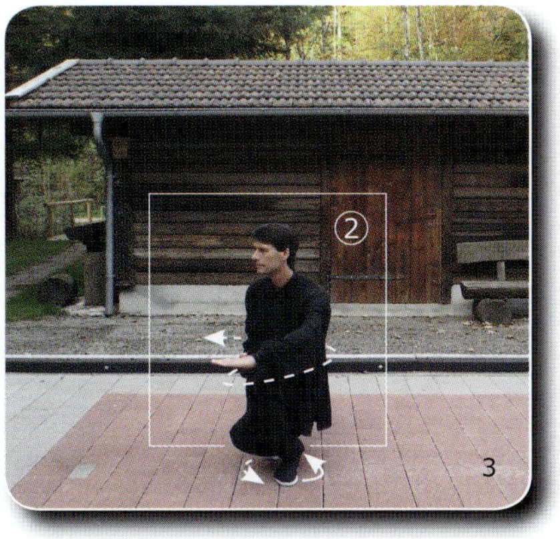


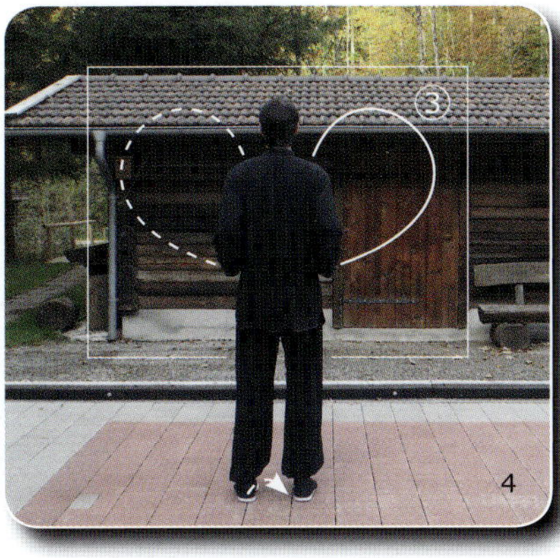


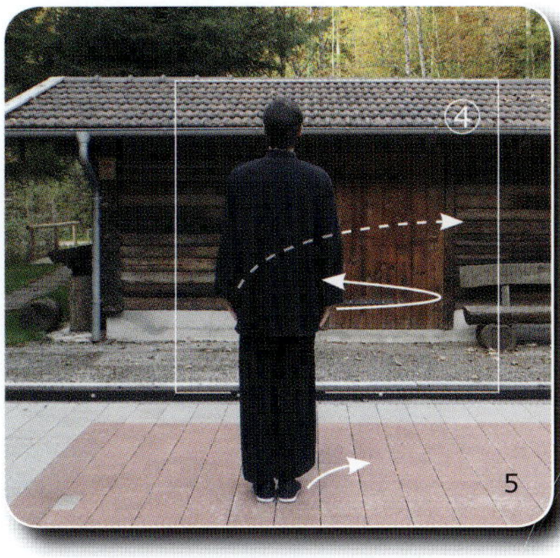


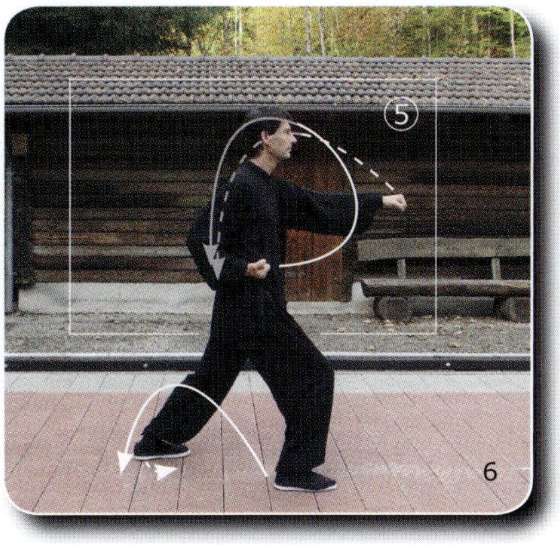


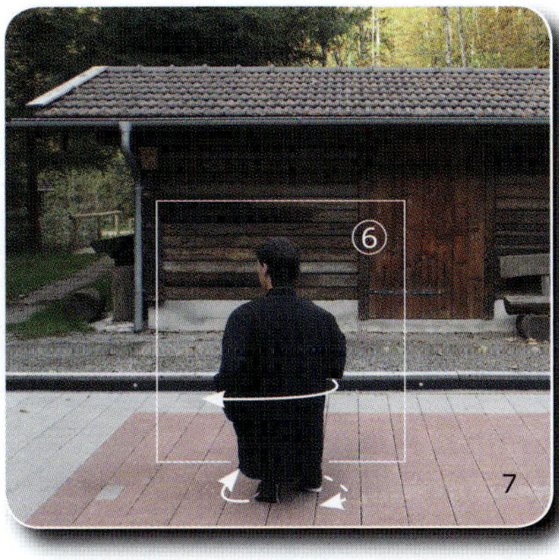


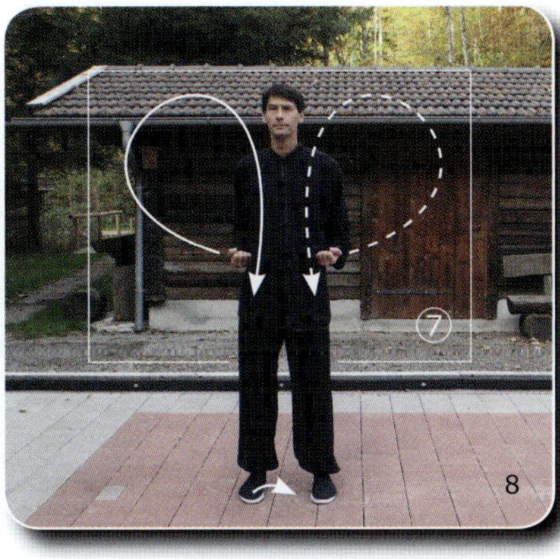


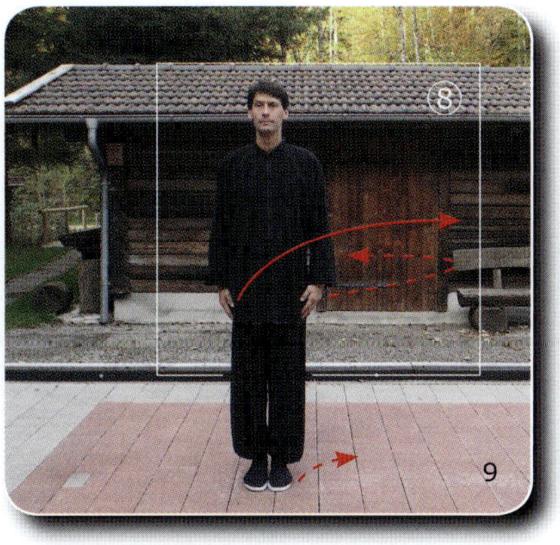

## 八、孔雀开屏
## VIII. Der Pfau öffnet seine Flügel und schlägt das Rad
## VIII. The Peacock Opens Its Wings and Spreads Its Tail

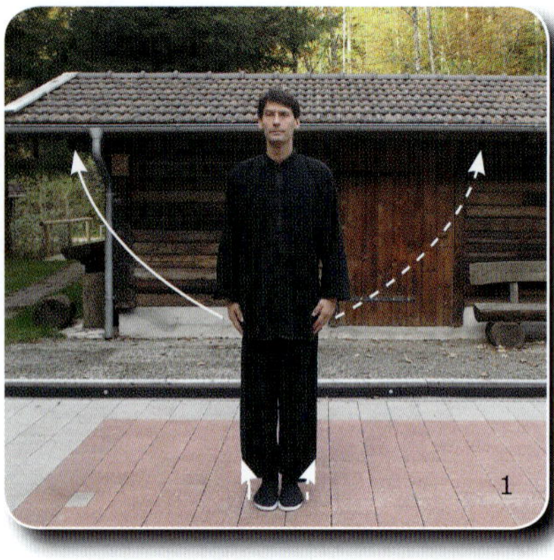


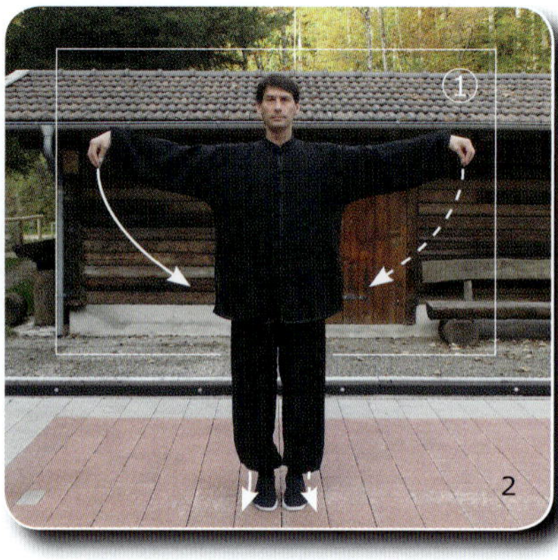


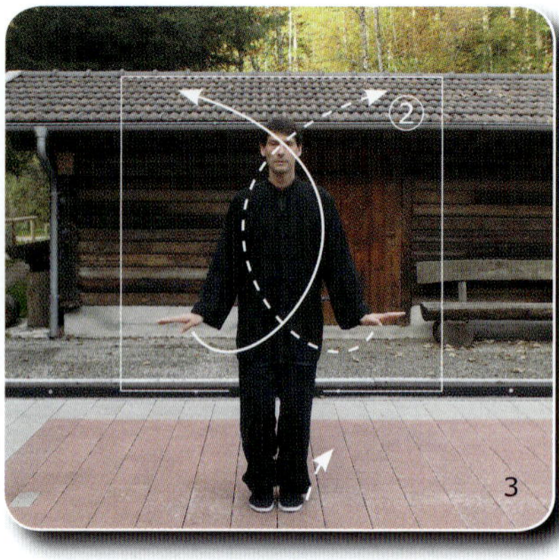


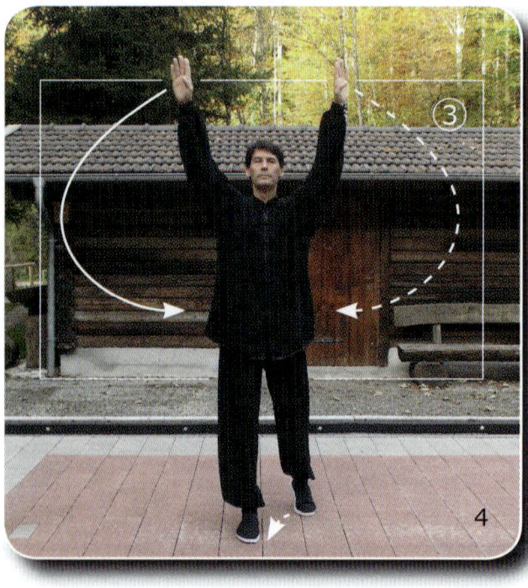


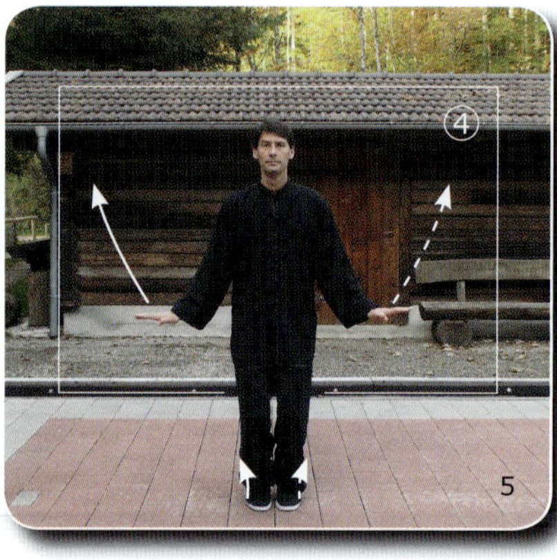


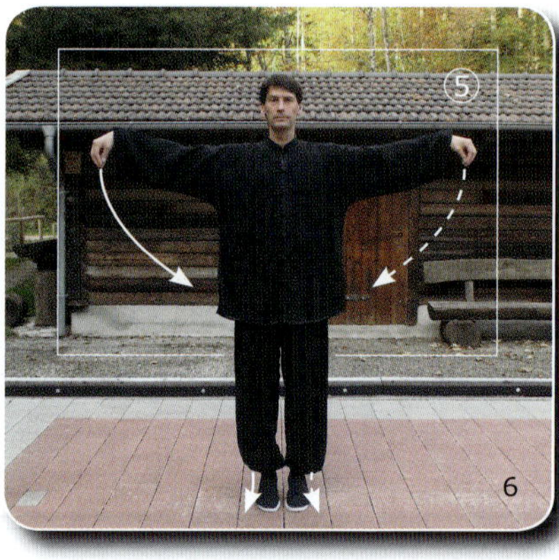


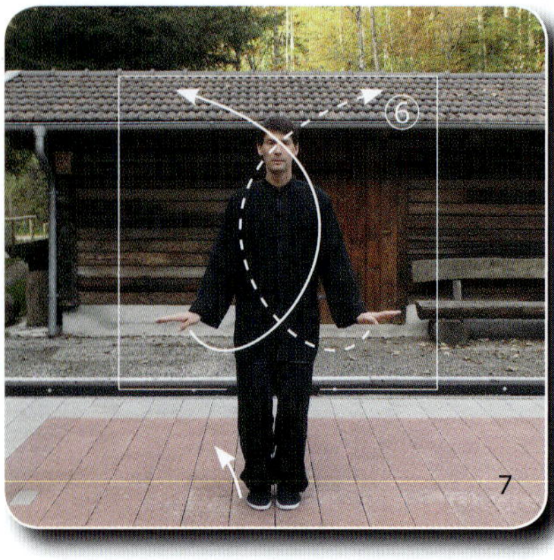


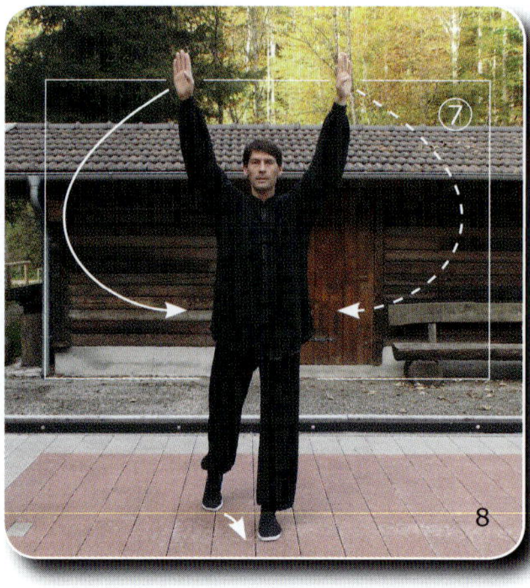


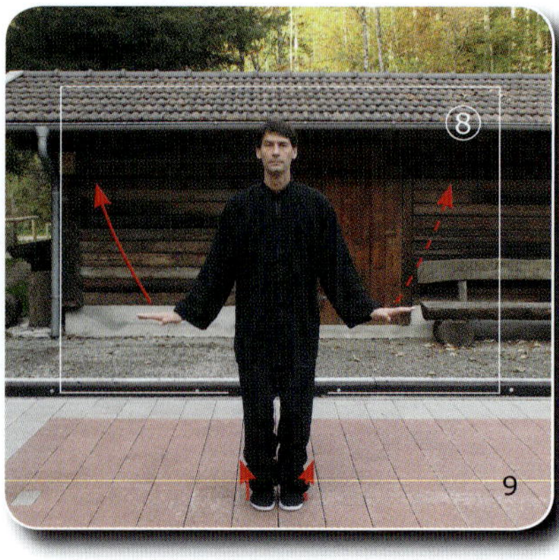

## 九、踏步展掌

## IX. Auf der Stelle treten und die Hände öffnen

## IX. Step at the Same Spot and Open Your Hands

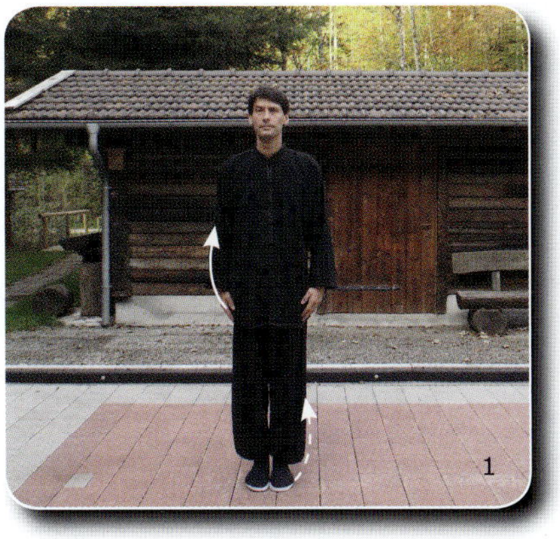
1

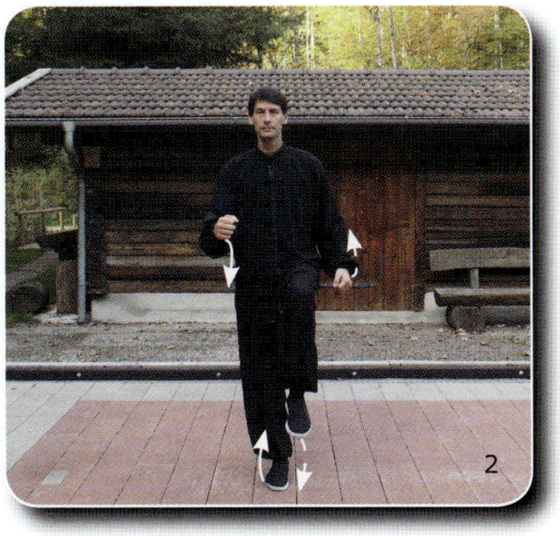
2

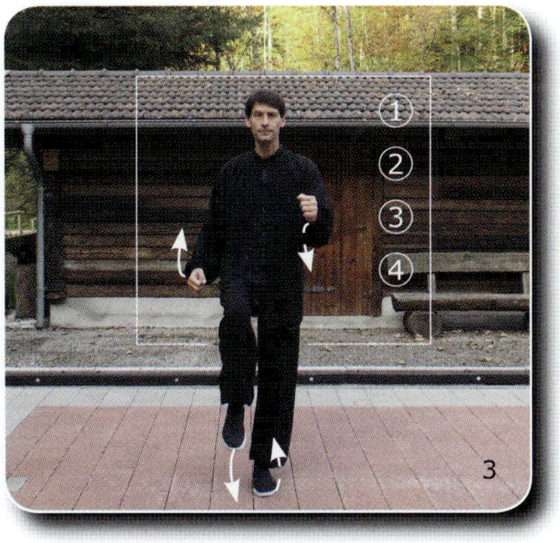

3

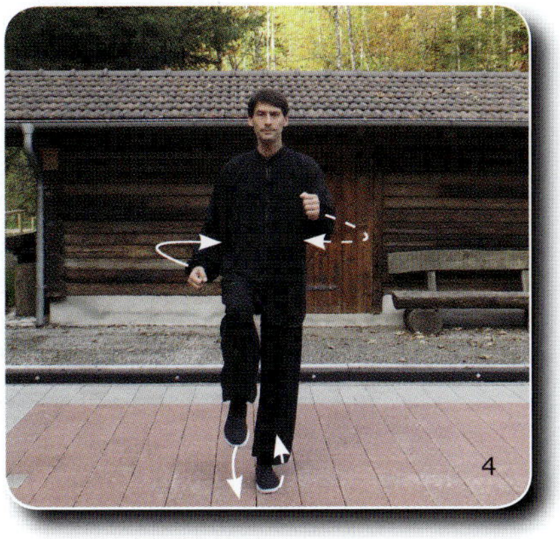
4

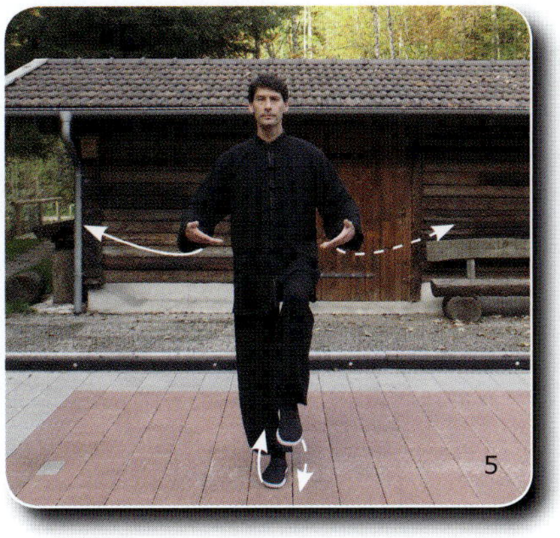
5

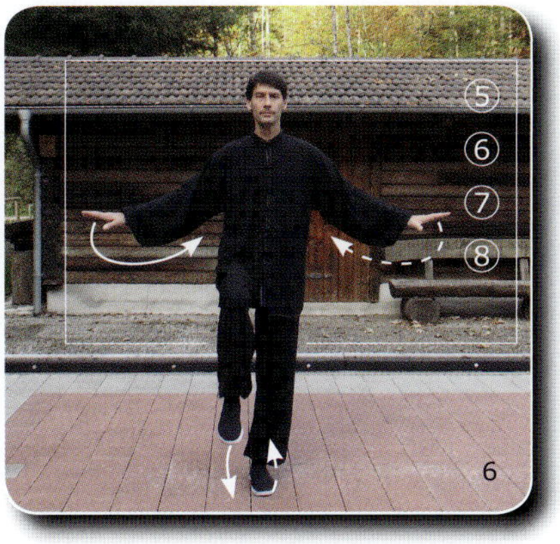

6

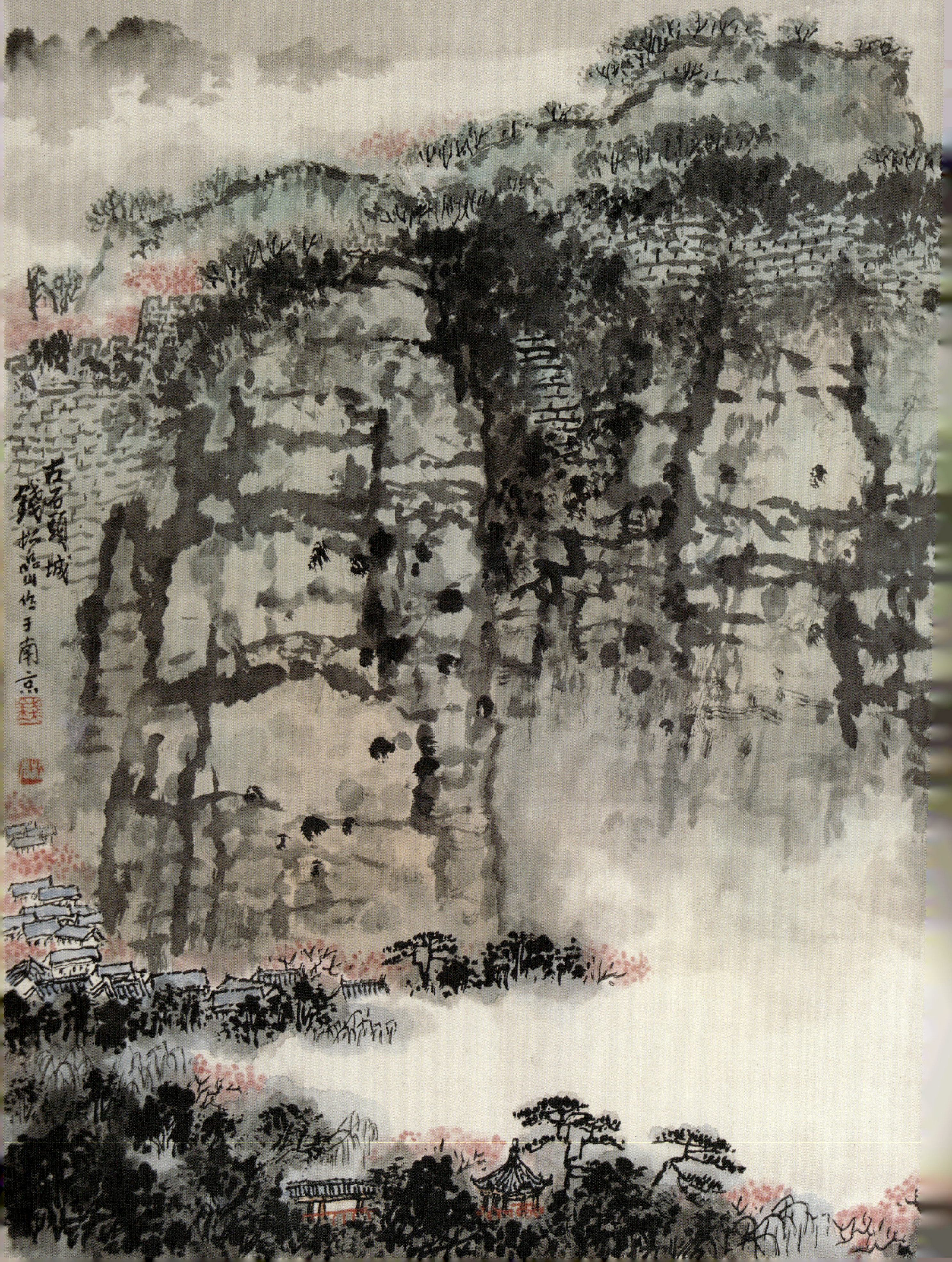
古石頭城
錢松喦作于南京

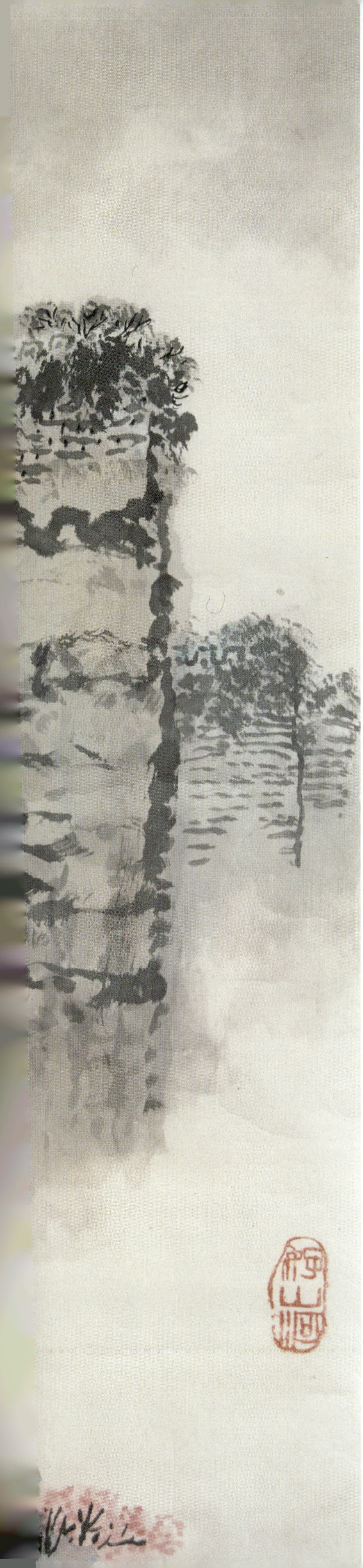

“古石头城”。钱松岩作于1960年。南京古称“石头城”、“金陵”。钱松岩出生于1899年9月，是20世纪中国最重要的画家之一。江苏宜兴人，曾任江苏省国画院院长、江苏省美术家协会主席，中国美术家协会常务理事、顾问，第四、五、六届全国人大代表，是当代中国山水画主要代表人之一。出版的个人画集（包括指画集）、理论著作过100集，拍摄专题纪录片3部。中国美术馆、人民大会堂、毛主席纪念堂、钓鱼台国宾馆均收藏或在显著位置陈列其作品。华国锋、胡耀邦、邓小平等国家领导人将其作品以国礼馈赠给法国总统、日本首相及著名的外国要人收藏。钱松岩的作品，章法构图变化多端，色彩运用大胆独特，个人风格显著明了，堪称“承前启后，一代宗师”。钱松岩于1985年9月在南京逝世。

„Alte Steinstadt“ wurde von Qian SongYan im Jahr 1960 gemalt. Die Stadt NanJing wurde früher „ShiTou Cheng“ („Alte Steinstadt“) oder „JinLing“ („Goldener Hügel“) genannt. Qian SongYan wurde im Jahr 1899 geboren und war im 20. Jahrhundert einer der bedeutendsten Maler Chinas. Er lehrte an verschiedenen Kunstakademien und war Direktor der Akademie für chinesische Malerei in der Provinz JiangSu. Seine Malerei, sowohl im traditionellen Stil als auch in dem von ihm entwickelten neuen kreativen Stil, wurde in zahlreichen Ausstellungen im In- und Ausland bekannt. Seine Bilder wurden von mehreren bekannten Museen gesammelt, z.B. vom Guggenheim Museum in New York. Sein Werk (u.a. auch Fingermalerei) wurde in über hundert Bänden herausgegeben. Qian SongYan starb im Jahr 1985 in NanJing.

"Old Town of Stone" was painted by Qian SongYan in 1960. In former times the city of NanJing was called "ShiTou Cheng" ("Old Town of Stone") or "JinLing" ("Golden Hill"). Qian SongYan was born in 1899 and was one of the most important painters in China. He taught at various academies of art and was director of the Academy for Chinese Painting in the province of JiangSu. His painting in the traditional style as well as in the new creative style developed by him became well-known in many exhibitions in China and abroad. His paintings were collected by several noted museums, so by the Guggenheim Museum in New York among others. His opus (including fingerpaintings) was published in more than a hundred volumes. Qian SongYan died in NanJing in 1985.

www.yan-gronau.de

# 附录

## 一、手式

1. 八字
手指打开如一个八字。（图1）

2. 勾手
大拇指轻轻扣着中指尖的指肚，其余三指慢慢合拢，掌心空开，五指间留有缝隙，掌心空开使五指自然的聚在一起。（图2）

3. 虎口
在手背拇、食指之间，即合谷穴。（图3）

4. 拳
（图4）

5. 掌
（图5）

1

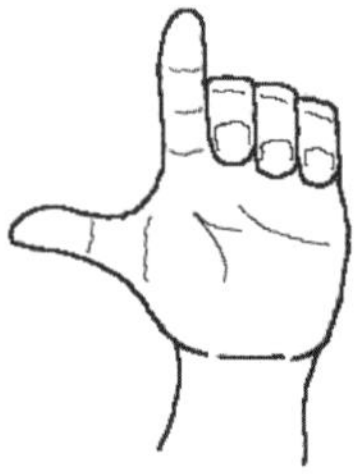

2

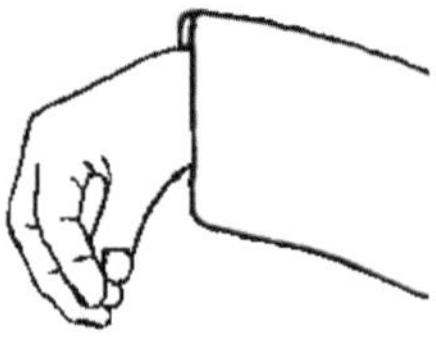

3

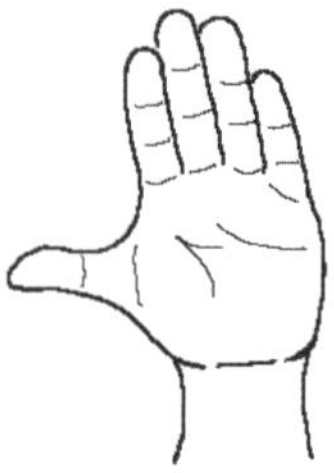

4

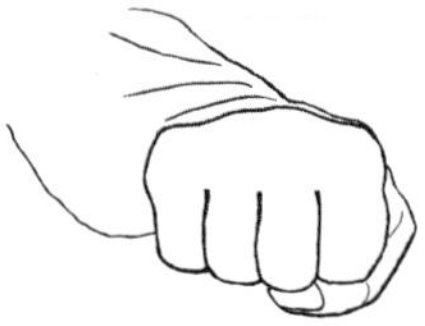

5

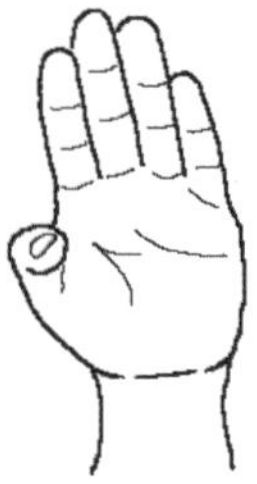

# Anhang

## I. Handhaltungen

1. BaZi 八字 Chinesisches Zeichen für die Acht
Handhaltung, bei der der Daumen vom gestreckten Zeigefinger weggespreizt wird. Die restlichen Finger werden am zweiten Fingerglied eingerollt.

2. GouShou 勾手 Hakenhand
Die Fingerspitzen des Daumens und der Finger werden zusammengebracht und das Handgelenk wird nach unten gebeugt.

3. HuKou 虎口 Tigermaul
Position der Hand mit gestreckten Fingern und rechtwinkelig abgespreiztem Daumen.

4. Quan 拳 Faust
Finger einrollen und den Daumen über die mittleren Fingerglieder legen. Handrücken und Unterarm sind auf einer Linie.

5. Zhang 掌 Handfläche
Position der Hand mit gestreckten Fingern, bei der der Daumen nach innen geknickt und eng am Handteller angelegt wird.

# Appendix

## I. Hand Positions

1. BaZi 八字 Chinese sign for eight
Handposition in which your thumb is spread off your forefinger in a right angle. Roll in your other fingers at your second knuckle-joint.

2. GouShou 勾手 Hookhand
The tips of your thumb and of your fingers are put together and your wrist is bent down.

3. HuKou 虎口 Mouth of the Tiger
Handposition with your fingers stretched straight and with your thumb spread off in a right angle.

4. Quan 拳 Fist
Roll in your fingers and put your thumb across your middle fingerjoints. The back of your hand and your forearm form one line.

5. Zhang 掌 Palm
Handposition with your fingers stretched straight and your thumb folded inside and put closely to your palm.

## 二、基本步形

1. 弓步

一腿全脚着地，屈膝前弓，承身体重量的三分之二，另一腿自然伸直，承身体重量的三分之一。（图1）

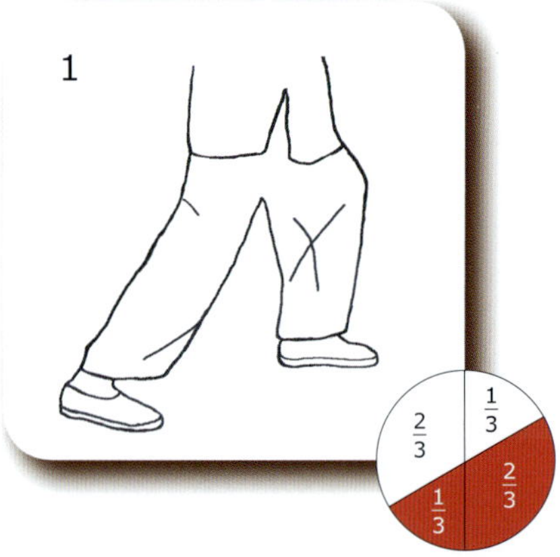


2. 开立步

图2中的姿势是开立步的一种。既两脚开立的距离略大于肩宽，身体重量均匀落于两脚。（图2）

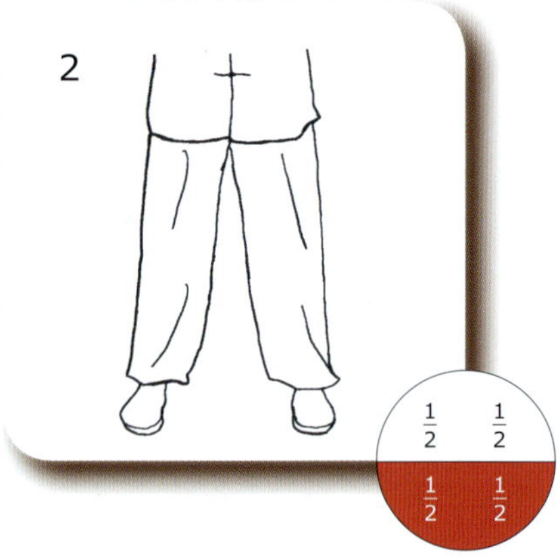


3. 马步

两脚开立下蹲，身体重量均匀落于两腿，两膝弯曲和脚尖朝同一方向。（图3）

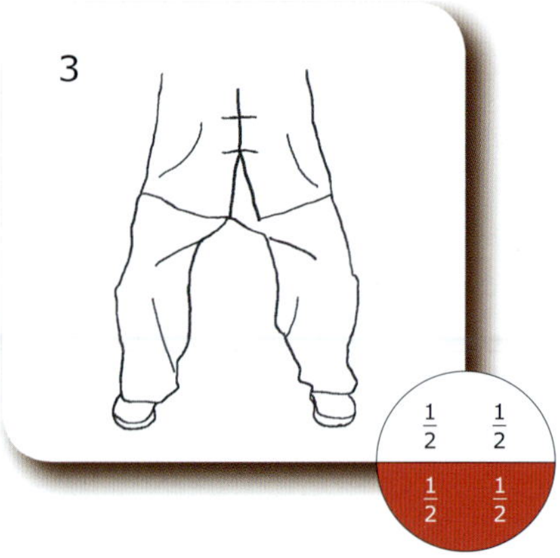


4. 歇步

两腿交叉靠拢全蹲，右脚全脚着地，脚尖外展，左脚前脚掌着地，膝部靠于前小腿外侧，臀部接于左脚跟处。（图4）

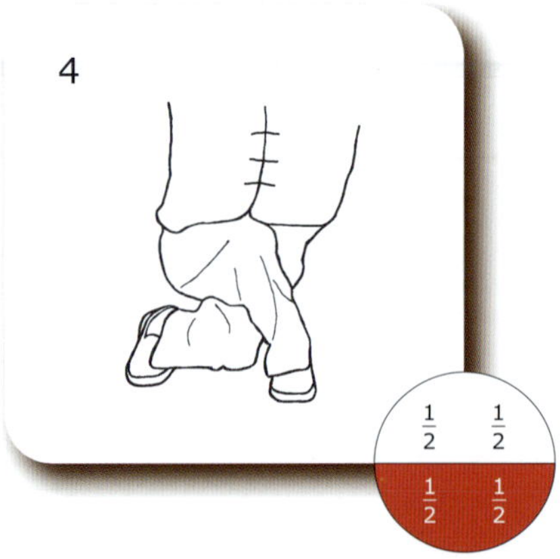


5. 虚步

一腿屈膝支承身体重量的约十分之八，另一腿微屈，脚尖点地向前，承身体重量的约十分之二。支撑腿和另一腿成30度。（图5）

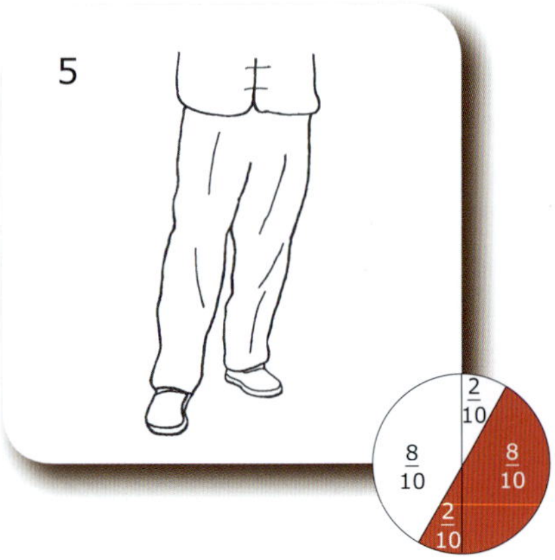

## II. Fußstellungen

1. GongBu 弓步 Bogenschritt
Das Körpergewicht befindet sich zu zwei Dritteln auf dem gebeugten Bein und zu einem Drittel auf dem gestreckten Bein. Das hintere Bein steht in einem Winkel von 45° zum vorderen Bein.

2. KaiLiBu 开立步 Schulterbreiter Stand
Das Körpergewicht ist gleichmäßig auf beide Füße verlagert.

3. MaBu 马步 Pferdeschritt
Bei dieser Position ist das Körpergewicht gleichmäßig auf beide Beine verlagert und die Knie sind gebeugt. Die Fußspitzen zeigen in dieselbe Richtung wie die Knie.

4. XieBu 歇步 Ruhender Schritt
Bei dieser Stellung geht man mit überkreuzten Beinen in die Hocke. Bei einem rechten XieBu berührt der rechte (vordere) Fuß mit der ganzen Fußsohle den Boden. Die Fußspitze ist dabei leicht nach außen gerichtet. Der linke Fuß ruht auf dem Ballen, das Knie drückt sich an die Außenseite des rechten Unterschenkels. Das Gesäß nähert sich der Ferse des linken Fußes. Das Gewicht ist etwa gleichmäßig auf beide Beine verteilt und der Oberkörper bleibt aufrecht.

5. XuBu 虚步 Leerer Schritt
Das Körpergewicht befindet sich zu acht Zehnteln auf dem gestreckten Bein und zu zwei Zehnteln auf dem anderen Bein. Die Ferse wird bei dem Bein, das weniger belastet ist, vom Boden gelöst. Der Fuß bleibt gerade nach vorne gerichtet. Das Bein, das das Körpergewicht zum Großteil trägt, steht in einem Winkel von 30° zum anderen Bein.

## II. Foot Positions

1. GongBu 弓步 Bow Stance
Your bodyweight is on the bent leg by two thirds, on the stretched leg by on third. Your backward leg forms an angle of 45° to your foremost leg.

2. KaiLiBu 开立步 Stance of Shoulder-Breadth
Your bodyweight is shifted on both feet equally.

3. MaBu 马步 Horse-Stance
In this position your bodyweight is shifted on both legs equally and the knees are bent. The tips of your feet have the same direction as your knees.

4. XieBu 歇步 Resting Stance
In this position you cross your legs in squatting down. In a right hand side XieBu your right (foremost) foot touches the ground with the complete sole of your foot. The tip of your foot is directed slighlty outwards in doing so. Your left foot rests on its ball, your knee presses onto the outside of your right shank. Your buttocks go near the heel of your left foot. Your bodyweight is approximately shifted onto both legs equally.

5. XuBu 虚步 Empty Stance
Your bodyweight is on your stretched leg by 8 tenths and on the other leg by 2 tenths. The leg which bears less weight detaches its heel off the ground. Your foot remains directed straight forward. The leg which bears most of your bodyweight has an angle of 30° to the other leg.

## 三、词汇注释表

### 八段锦

八段锦是中国传统保健功法。古人把这套动作比喻为“锦”，意为动作舒展优美，如锦缎般优美、柔顺，又因为功法共为八段，每段一个动作，故名为“八段锦”。

### 寸

10寸等于1尺，1寸约合3.33厘米，1米=30寸。

### 带脉

带脉是人体奇经八脉之一。带脉在人体的腰部围一圈，是一条横向的经脉。人体上其它的经脉都是纵向的，这条经脉就好像一条绳子将所有的经脉系在一起，所以称为带脉。

### 丹田

分上丹田、中丹田和下丹田。上丹田在头顶百会穴，有说在两眉间印堂穴。中丹田在胸部膻中穴，有说巨阙穴。下丹田在脐下小腹部分，包括关元、气海，神阙、命门等穴位。（图1）

### 大椎穴

督脉穴，在后背部正中线上，第7颈椎棘突下凹陷中。（图2）

### 风池穴

在头额后面大筋的两旁与耳垂平行处。胆经气血在此吸热后化为阳热风气。（图3）

1

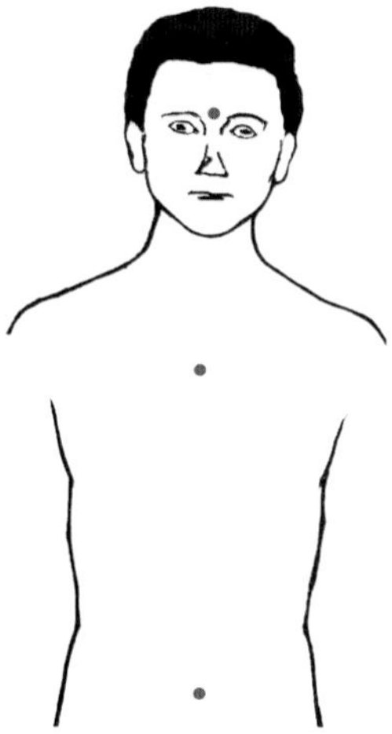

2

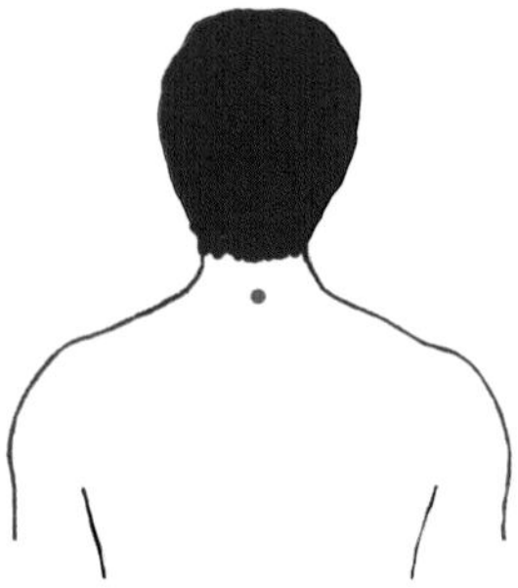

3

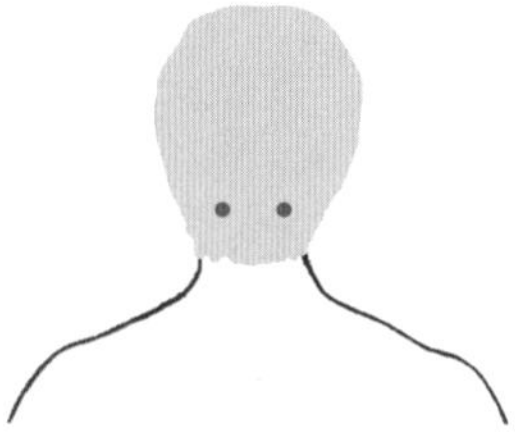

## III. Erklärungen

BaDuanJin 八段锦 bedeutet wörtlich übersetzt „Acht Stücke Brokat". BaDuanJin ist eine klassische Fitness-Übung, bestehend aus acht Übungen.

Cun 寸 Traditionelle chinesische Maßeinheit
Definiert ein Zehntel eines chinesischen Fußes (Chi). In der Volksrepublik China wurde das Chi 1984 auf 0,33 Meter festgelegt. Ein Cun hat 3,33 cm.

DaiMai 带脉 Gürtelgefäß
Dai bedeutet Gürtel und Mai Gefäß. Es befindet sich an der Taille.

DanTian 丹田 Energiezentren
Man unterscheidet drei Energiezentren, das obere, mittlere und untere DanTian. Das obere DanTian befindet sich im Stirnbereich zwischen den Augenbrauen (beim YinTang Punkt). Das mittlere DanTian liegt in der Mitte des Brustbeins (beim ShanZhong Punkt), das untere DanTian ist im Bauchbereich, etwa 3,5 cm unterhalb des Nabels (beim GuanYuan Punkt). Diese Energiezentren befinden sich nicht an der Körperoberfläche. Siehe Bild 1.

DaZhui 大椎穴 Großer Wirbel
Der Punkt befindet sich im oberen Bereich des Rückens auf dem Lenkergefäß. Die chinesische Bezeichnung für diesen Meridian ist DuMai. Siehe Bild 2.

FengChi 风池穴 Windteich
Der Punkt befindet sich am Hinterkopf auf dem Gallenblasenmeridian. Die chinesische Bezeichnung für diesen Meridian ist DanJing. Siehe Bild 3.

## III. Explanations

BaDuanJin 八段锦 means "Eight Pieces of Brocade" in literal translation. BaDuanJin is a classical fitness exercise consisting of eight exercises.

Cun 寸 Traditional Chinese measurement
Defines one tenth of a Chinese foot (Chi). In the People´s Republic of China one Chi was fixed at 0,33 metres in 1984. One Cun has 3,33 centimetres.

DaiMai 带脉 Belt Meridian
Dai means belt und Mai means vessel. It is situated at your waist.

DanTian 丹田 Centres of Energy
You distinguish 3 energy-centres, the upper, middle and inferior DanTian. The upper DanTian is situated in the region of the forehead between the eyebrows (at YinTang Point). The middle DanTian is situated in the the middle of the breastbone (at ShanZhong Point), and the inferior DanTian is in the area of the abdomen, about 3,5 cm beneath the navel (at GuanYuan Point). These centres of energy are not situated on the surface of the body. See illustration 1.

DaZhui 大椎穴 Big Vertebra
The point is situated in the upper region of the back on the Leader Vessel. The Chinese name of this channel is DuMai. See illustration 2.

FengChi 风池穴 Wind Pool
The point is situated on the back of your head on the Gall Bladder Channel. The Chinese name of the channel is DanJing. See illustration 3.

环跳穴

经穴名，属足少阳胆经。足少阳、太阳之会。在股外侧部，侧卧屈股，当股骨大转子最凸点与骶管裂孔连线的外三分之一与中三分之一交点处。（图4）

4

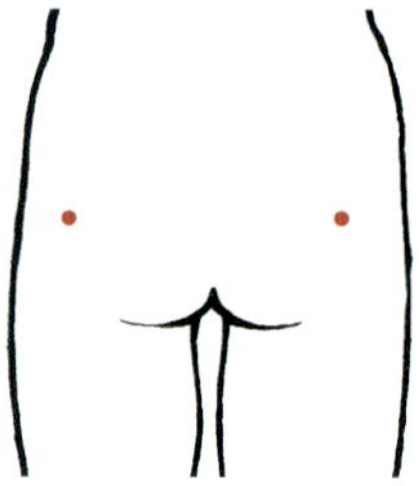

筋骨功

气功功法，共9 个动作，可强筋健骨。

劳宫穴

经穴名，属手厥阴心包经穴，位于人体的手掌心，在握拳屈指时无名指尖处。因“手任劳作，穴在掌心”而定名为劳宫穴。（图5）

5

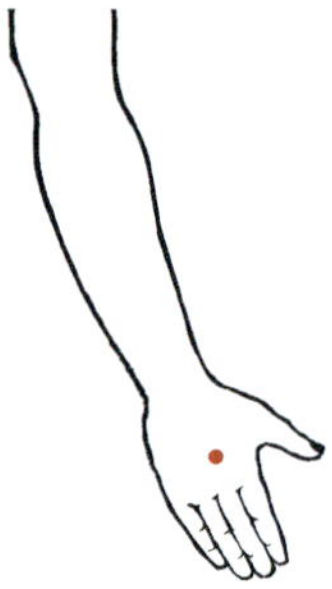

米

在练习功法时以米字格来规范动作。

命门穴

命，人之根本。门，出入的门户。命门穴位于人体的腰部，当后正中线上，第二腰椎棘突下凹陷处。经属督脉。指压时，有强烈的压痛感。（图6）

6

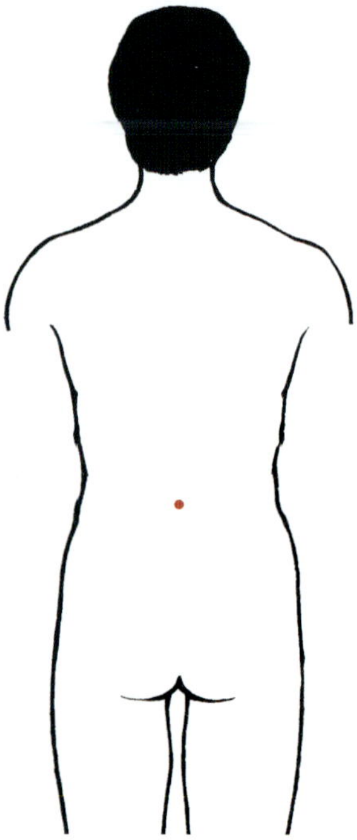

内经

《黄帝内经》简称《内经》，是中国现存医书中最早的典籍之一。《黄帝内经》是一部综合论述中医理论的经典著作。它的成书是以古代的解剖知识为基础，通过对生命现象的长期观察，以及医疗实践的反复验证，逐渐发展而成的。《黄帝内经》为古代医者托黄帝之名所作。之所以冠以“黄帝”之名，意在溯源崇本，藉以说明书中所言非虚。

气

是太极和气功及中医中常见的概念。天地一切事物组成的基本元素，有着像气体般的流动特性。人类与一切生物具备的生命能量或动力，也被称为是气。中医学认为气是人体的第一道防护线，聚于体里保护着五脏六腑，散发于肤表以防外邪侵入而导致疾病发生。

HuanTiao 环跳穴 Zurückspringen
Der Punkt befindet sich am Gesäß auf dem Gallenblasenmeridian. Die chinesische Bezeichnung für diesen Meridian ist DanJing. Siehe Bild 4.

JinGu Gong 筋骨功 QiGong Form
Jin sind die Sehnen und Gu die Knochen. Form des QiGong, bestehend aus neun Übungen. Der Schwerpunkt der Übung ist darauf gerichtet, die Sehnen zu ziehen und zu dehnen sowie die Knochen zu stabilisieren.

LaoGong 劳宫穴 Palast der Arbeit
Dieser Punkt befindet sich in der Mitte der Handfläche auf dem Perikardmeridian. Die chinesische Bezeichnung für diesen Meridian ist XinBao. Siehe Bild 5.

Mi 米 Reis

MingMen 命门穴 Tor des Lebens
Dieser Punkt liegt im Bereich des unteren Rückens auf dem Lenkergefäß. Die chinesische Bezeichnung für diesen Meridian ist DuMai. Siehe Bild 6.

NeiJing 内经 Kanon der Inneren Medizin
Medizinisches Fachwerk, das bis heute grundlegend und richtungweisend für die Ausbildung innerhalb der Traditionellen Chinesischen Medizin ist. Das NeiJing ist eine Sammlung von 81 Abhandlungen, die aus zwei Teilen besteht. Der erste Teil ist zur Zeit von HuangDi, des mythischen Gelben Kaisers (2696 - 2598 v. Chr.), erschienen.

Qi 气 Luft, Atem, Lebensenergie

HuanTiao 环跳穴 Backjump
The point is situated on the buttocks on the Gall Bladder Channel. The Chinese name of the channel is DanJing. See illustration 4.

JinGu Gong 筋骨功 Form of QiGong
Jin are the sinews and Gu the bones. Form of QiGong consisting of nine exercises. The crucial point of the exercise aims at drawing and stretching the sinews as well as stabilizing the bones.

LaoGong 劳宫穴 Palace of Work
This point is situated in the middle of your palm at the Pericardial Meridian. The Chinese name of this meridian is XinBao. See illustration 5.

Mi 米 Rice

MingMen 命门穴 Gate of Life
This point is situated in the region of the nether back on the Leader Vessel. The Chinese name of this meridian is DuMai. See illustration 6.

NeiJing 内经 Canon of internal medicine
Medical work which is fundamental and leading for the study of Traditional Chinese Medicine. NeiJing is a collection of 81 treatises consisting of two parts. The first part was published at the time of HungDi, the mythical Yellow Emperor (2696 - 2598 B. C.).

Qi 气 Air, breath, energy of life

气功

通过以呼吸的调整、身体活动的调整和意识的调整（调息，调形，调心）为锻炼方法，务求达到强身健体、健康身心、抗病延年等目的。

七伤

大饱伤脾，大怒气逆伤肝，强力举重久坐湿地伤肾，形寒饮冷伤肺，形劳意损伤神，风雨寒暑伤形，恐惧不节伤志。五劳七伤，泛指各种疾病和致病因素。人们经常用“五劳七伤”来形容人身体虚弱多病。

肾俞穴

足太阳膀胱经穴。在腰部，当第2腰椎棘突下，旁开1.5寸。肾脏的寒湿水气由此外输膀胱经。（图7）

五劳

久视伤血，久卧伤气，久坐伤肉，久立伤骨，久行伤筋，是谓五劳所伤。五劳七伤，泛指各种疾病和致病因素。人们经常用“五劳七伤”来形容人身体虚弱多病。

胃经

足阳明胃经。简称胃经。人体十二经脉之一，是从头部开始，经脖子、胸、腹、下肢以至足尖等非常长的经脉。有很多对消化系统非常重要的穴位。（图8）

7

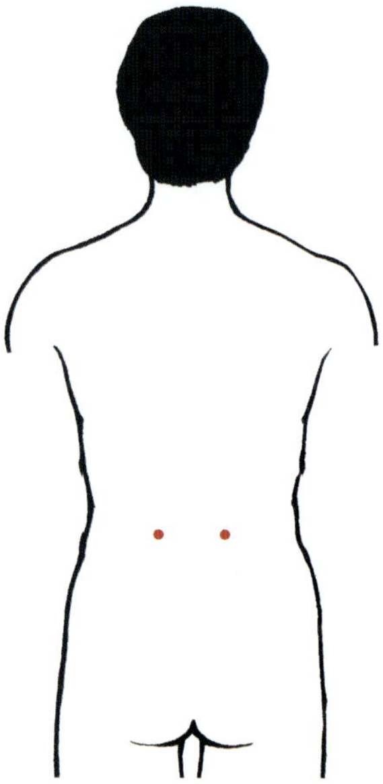

8

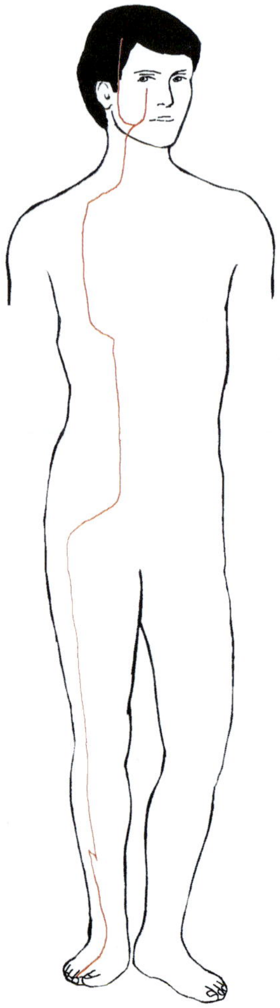

QiGong 气功 Atemübungen

QiShang 七伤 Die Sieben Betrübnisse[1]
1. Zu viel Essen schädigt die Milz;
2. Wut schädigt die Leber (Wut ändert die Richtung, in der die Energie (Qi) normal läuft);
3. Starke körperliche Anstrengungen und langes Sitzen schädigen die Nieren;
4. Kalte Getränke schädigen die Lunge;
5. Sorgen schädigen die Nerven;
6. Wind, Regen, Kälte im Winter und Hitze im Sommer schädigen den Körper;
7. Zu viel Angst schädigt Moral und Standhaftigkeit.

ShenShu 肾俞穴 Transportpunkt zu den Nieren
Dieser Punkt befindet sich am Rücken auf dem Blasenmeridian. Die chinesiche Bezeichnung für diesen Meridian ist PangGuangJing. Siehe Bild 7.

WuLao 五劳 Die Fünf Anstrengungen (durch den Einfluß von Müdigkeit)[1]
1. Langes Sehen (Lesen) schädigt das Blut;
2. Langes Liegen schädigt die Lebensenergie (Qi);
3. Langes Sitzen schädigt das Fleisch (Muskeln);
4. Langes Stehen schädigt die Knochen;
5. Langes Laufen schädigt die Sehnen.

WeiJing 胃经 Magenmeridian
Siehe Bild 8.

[1] In der Fachsprache der Traditionellen Chinesischen Medizin stehen die Fünf Anstregungen und die Sieben Betrübnisse für eine Vielzahl von Krankheiten, Risikofaktoren und Ursachen für Krankheiten.

QiGong 气功 Breathing Exercises

QiShang 七伤 Seven Afflictions[1]
1. Too much food harms your spleen;
2. Rage harms your liver (rage changes the direction in which energy (Qi) normally runs);
3. Great bodily stress and longtime sitting harm your kidneys;
4. Cold beverages harm your lungs;
5. Worrying harms your nerves;
6. Wind, rain, cold in winter and heat in summer harm your body;
7. Too much fear harms your morals and steadfastness.

ShenShu 肾俞穴 Transport Point leading to your kidneys
This point is situated on your back at the Bladder Meridian. Its Chinese name is Pang GuangJing. See illustration 7.

WuLao 五劳 Five Strains (by the influrence of tiredness)[1]
1. Longtime watching (reading) harms your blood;
2. Longtime lying harms your energy of life (Qi);
3. Longtime sitting harms your flesh (muscles);
4. Longtime standing harms your bones;
5. Longtime walking harms your sinews.

WeiJing 胃经 Stomach Channel
See illustration 8.

[1] In the idiom of Traditional Chinese Medicine the Five Strains and Seven Afflictions stand for a great number of illnesses, risk factors and causes of illnesses.

意守/意在

意守是气功常用术语。意，指意识、意念或精神。守，指集中和保持住。意守通常是指气功锻炼过程中，将意念集中和保持在身体某一部位，或某一事物上的方法和过程。通过意守，可以帮助排除杂念。

涌泉穴

涌，外涌而出也。泉，泉水也。该穴名意指体内肾经的经水由此外涌而出体表。涌泉穴为肾经经脉的第一穴，它联通肾经的体内体表经脉，位于足底部。（图9）

足三里

足三里穴是足阳明胃经的主要穴位之一，位于小腿外侧。（图10）

9

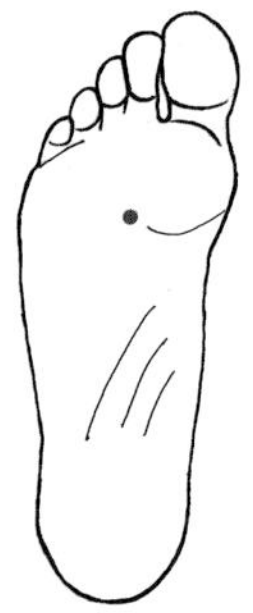

10

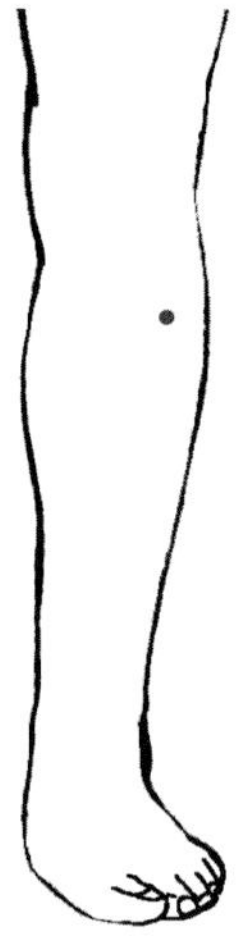

YiShou/YiZai 意守/意在 Vorstellungskraft
Ein wichtiger Aspekt bei den Übungen des QiGong ist die Arbeit mit der Vorstellungskraft. Man versucht durch die Konzentration des Geistes die Aufmerksamkeit auf bestimmte Punkte bzw. Energiezentren zu fokussieren.

YongQuan 涌泉穴 Sprudelnde Quelle
Dieser Punkt befindet sich auf dem Nierenmeridian, auf der Fußsohle. Die chinesische Bezeichnung für diesen Meridian ist ShenJing. Siehe Bild 9.

ZuSanLi 足三里 Drei Meilen am Bein
Dieser Punkt befindet sich etwas unterhalb des Knies auf dem Magenmeridian. Die chinesische Bezeichnung für diesen Meridian ist WeiJing. Siehe Bild 10.



YiShou/YiZai 意守/意在 Power of Imagination
One important aspect with regard to QiGong exercises is the work with your power of imagination. By concentrating your mind you try to focus your attention on certain points or centres of energy.

YongQuan 涌泉穴 Bubbling Spring
This point is situated on the Kidney Channel on the sole of your foot. The Chinese name of this meridian is ShenJing.
See illustration 9.

ZuSanLi 足三里 Three Miles on Your Leg
This point is situated somewhat beneath your knee on the Stomach Channel. The Chinese name of this meridian is WeiJing.
See illustration 10.

活得健康，丁宏余
LILIOM 出版社，德国 Waging am See，2016，精装版，中、德、英三种语言

Professor Ding HongYu, Lebe die Gesundheit
LILIOM Verlag Waging am See (Deutschland) 2016, gebundene Ausgabe,
in drei Sprachen (Chinesisch, Deutsch und Englisch)

Professor Ding HongYu, Live Your Health
Published by LILIOM Waging am See (Germany) 2016, bound edition,
in three languages (Chinese, German and English)

ISBN 978-3-934785-76-2

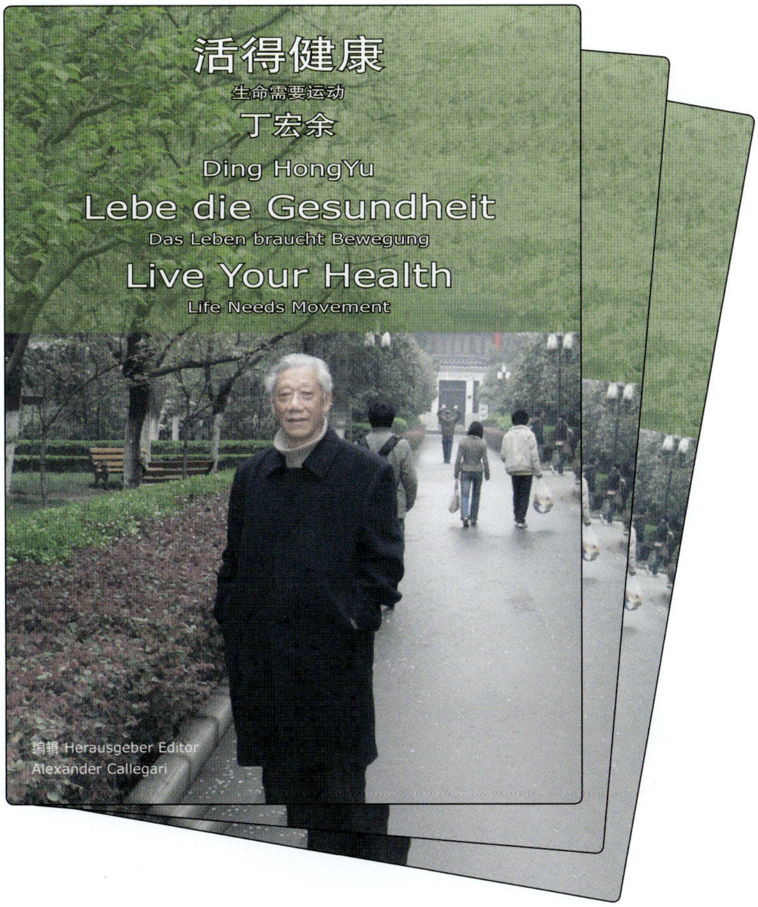


www.liliomverlag.de

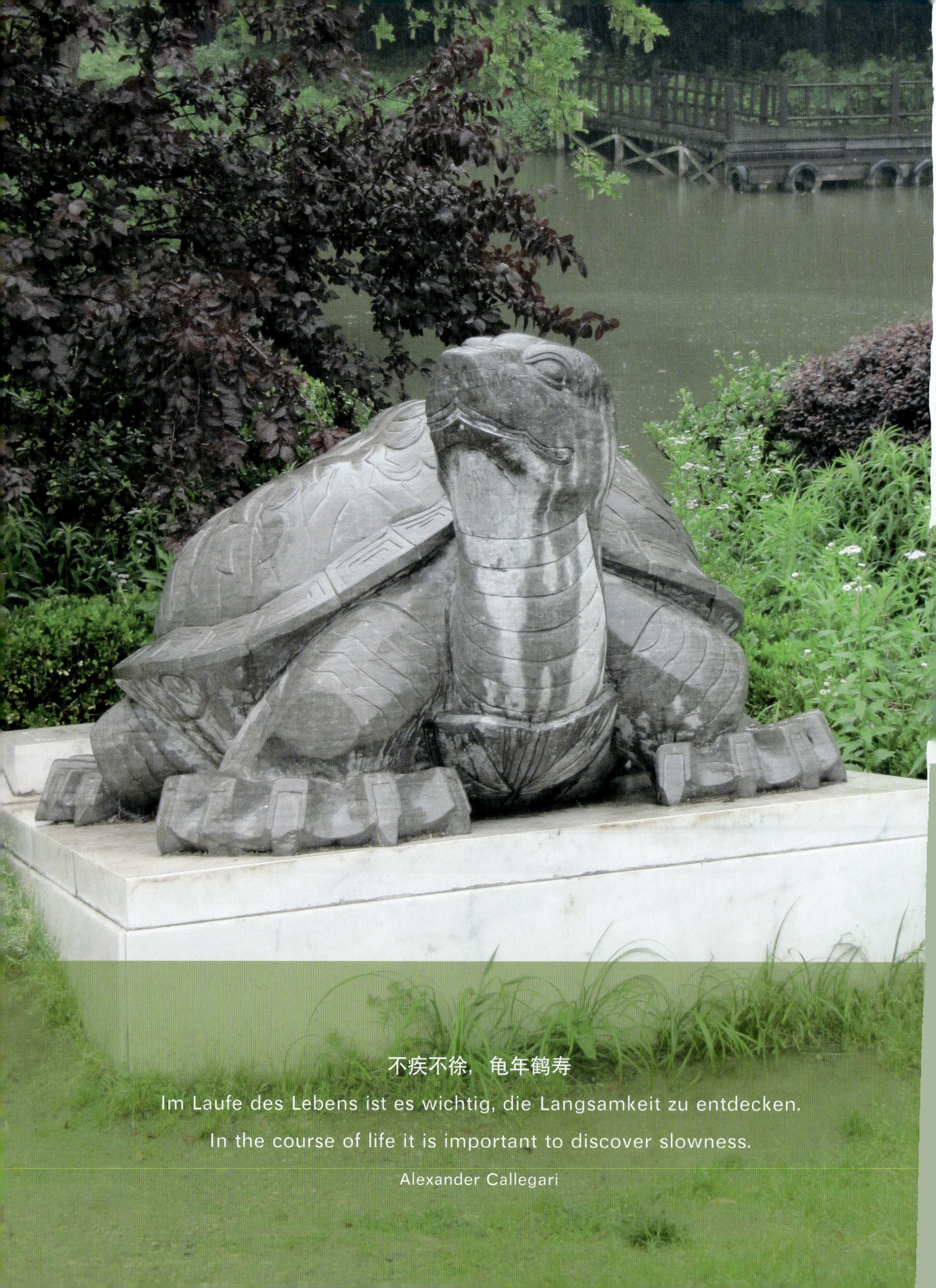

不疾不徐，龟年鹤寿

Im Laufe des Lebens ist es wichtig, die Langsamkeit zu entdecken.

In the course of life it is important to discover slowness.

Alexander Callegari